Addiction for Nurses

This book is dedicated to Yasmin Soraya, Adam Ali Hussein, Reshad Hassan, Leyla, Isra Oya, Mariam Safian and Hassim.

There is no wealth like knowledge, no poverty like ignorance.

Ali Ibn Abi Talib (RadiAllah Anhu)

Addiction for Nurses

Professor G. Hussein Rassool

PhD, MSc, BA, FRSPH, ILTM Cert. Ed., Cert. Couns., Cert. in Supervision and Consultation

Director of Inter-Cultural Therapy Centre, Mauritius
Visiting Professor of Addiction and Mental Health, Departamento de Psiquiatria e Ciências Humanas da Escola de Enfermagem de Ribeirão Preto da Universidade de São Paulo, Brazil
Visiting Professor, Federal University of Minas Gerais, Brazil
Florence Nightingale Research Foundation Scholar
Formerly Senior Lecturer in Addictive Behaviour, Department of Addictive Behaviour and Psychological Medicine, Centre for Addiction Studies, St George's University of London, UK

WILEY-BLACKWELL

A John Wiley & Sons, Ltd., Publication

Blackwell Publishing was acquired by John Wiley & Sons in February 2007. Blackwell's publishing programme has been merged with Wiley's global Scientific, Technical, and Medical business to form Wiley-Blackwell.

Registered office
John Wiley & Sons Ltd, The Atrium, Southern Gate, Chichester, West Sussex, PO19 8SQ, United Kingdom

Editorial offices
9600 Garsington Road, Oxford, OX4 2DQ, United Kingdom
2121 State Avenue, Ames, Iowa 50014-8300, USA

For details of our global editorial offices, for customer services and for information about how to apply for permission to reuse the copyright material in this book please see our website at www.wiley.com/wiley-blackwell.

The Library of Congress has cataloged the printed edition as follows:

Rassool, G. Hussein.
  Addiction for nurses / G. Hussein Rassool.
    p. ; cm.
  Includes bibliographical references and index.
  Summary: 'PRIMARY READERSHIP Student nurses (mental health branch) Postgraduate nursing students of addiction SECONDARY READERSHIP Addiction Nurses Community Nurses Mental Health Nurses'–Provided by publisher.
  ISBN 978-1-4051-8746-6 (pbk. : alk. paper) – ISBN 978-1-4443-2782-3 (e-book)   1. Substance abuse–Nursing.   2. Compulsive behavior–Nursing.   I. Title.
  [DNLM: 1. Substance-Related Disorders–nursing.   2. Behavior, Addictive–nursing. WY 160 R228a 2010]
  RC564.R356 2010
  616.86'0231–dc22

                                                                                    2010016814

A catalogue record for this book is available from the British Library.

Set in 10/12.5 pt Palatino by Toppan Best-set Premedia Limited
Printed and bound in Malaysia by Vivar Printing Sdn Bhd

1   2010

Contents

Preface

Addiction to alcohol and drugs is the foundation of this book. Alcohol and drug misuse is now regarded as a public health problem. The main aim is to promote understanding of the issues and strategies surrounding drug and alcohol use and misuse. It also aims to introduce nurses to the recognition, assessment, prevention and intervention strategies that can be used to support patients in their early identification and management of drugs and alcohol.

The book provides an overview of the approach to addiction and underpins a number of current policy initiatives as applied to current practice. It crystallises the nature of addiction, the health consequences of alcohol and drugs, and makes the complexity of the issues associated with addiction more accessible. It is designed to help nurses and generic health and social care professionals to understand the extent and nature of addiction and provides a framework to assist practitioners in working with alcohol and drug misusers. It provides a timely and practical introduction to the field of addiction.

Acknowledgments

I would like to thank all the staff at Wiley-Blackwell for their support and patience throughout the process of writing and publishing this book.

I am also particularly grateful to Professor Robert West, Addiction Press, who mooted the idea of writing a practical and no-nonsense book on addiction for nurses. To Emily Meir who gave me the opportunity to teach nurses. My thanks also go to Professor James P. Smith, Professor John Strang, Professor A. Hamid Ghodse and Dr. Nek Oyefeso for their guidance in my professional development. Special thanks go to Professor Margarita Villar-Luis, Escola De Enfermagem de Ribeirão Preto, Universidade de Sao Paulo, Brazil for our collaboration and development in publishing, teaching and research activities in addiction and mental health.

I am beholden to my patients and students for teaching me about practice in the addiction field. Thanks also go to all the 'Mousquetaires'-'Barbiers de Seville' and my brothers and sisters at Al-Furqaan, Les Guibies for their friendship and support. I would like to acknowledge the contributions of my teachers who enabled me, through my own reflective practices, to follow the path.

My special thanks also to Mariam for all the help and support during the writing of the book. Finally, I owe my gratitude to my family, Yasmin, Adam Reshad, Leyla and Isra for being here.

1 Introduction: Nursing Roles and Challenges

Nurses and other health care professionals form a core component of many health care systems so their roles in responding to the challenges set by the increase in the use of psychoactive substance use are crucial. Nurses in both primary health care and residential settings are usually the first point of contact with many who misuse alcohol and drugs. Nurses are often reluctant to work with alcohol and drug misusers, mainly because of anxieties concerning role adequacy, legitimacy and lack of support.

This chapter will examine the role of nurses in hospital and primary health care settings in relation to intervention and management of substance use and misuse. It will also look at the rationale for working with substance misusers, confidentiality and the contribution that nursing practice can provide.

Standards of conduct, performance and ethics for nurses and midwives

Nurses have a shared set of values, which find their expression in *The Code: standards of conduct, performance and ethics for nurses and midwives* (NMC 2007). Nurses have the following responsibilities:

Addiction for Nurses By G. Hussein Rassool. © 2010 G. Hussein Rassool

- To make the care of people their first concern, treating them as individuals and respecting their dignity.
- To work with others to protect and promote the health and wellbeing of those in their care, the patients' families and carers, and the wider community.
- To provide a high standard of practice and care at all times.
- To be open and honest, act with integrity and uphold the reputation of their profession.

Alcohol and drug misusers must be able to trust nurses with their health and wellbeing. The Code also states that 'as a professional, you are personally accountable for actions and omissions in your practice and must always be able to justify your decisions' and that 'you must always act lawfully, whether those laws relate to your professional practice or personal life'. Those with early substance use problems, chronic problem drinkers and drug users have the same rights *vis-à-vis* other patients in receiving appropriate health care from the National Health Service (NHS). Every member of the health care profession has an important role to play in responding to substance misuse problems.

The need to work with substance misusers

Given the extent and nature of the normalisation of psychoactive substances in society, only a minority of drug and alcohol misusers is likely to come into contact with specialist drug and alcohol agencies. Most of them will invariably have first contact with primary care services, medical and psychiatric services, social services and voluntary agencies, and the criminal justice system. The need for the management and treatment of substance misuse problems is no longer confined to the specialist services. Nurses, in different specialities and settings, are also likely to come into contact with alcohol and drug misusers.

An early intervention in the lifestyle and behaviour of substance misusers helps to limit the associated health, social and familial harms (Rassool 2009). Early intervention strategies from health and social care professionals can have a dramatic impact on preventing substance misuse becoming a long-term problem. The management of those with established substance use problems and those at an early stage of use is not the sole responsibility of specialist workers and addiction specialists. An active involvement of the different cadres of health workers in managing problems of substance misuse is necessary because of the sharp increase, in recent times, in the number of users of psychoactive substances with abuse potential (Rassool & Oyefeso 1993).

A broad range of health, social work and criminal justice system workers have a key role to play in addressing substance misuse and the reduction of substance misuse should be regarded as a core business for many services. Every role in the drug and alcohol field requires a particular set of competences. Some of these will be generic, others more specific to the substance misuse field, and the required competences will vary from one role to another (Home Office 2005).

Table 1.1 Working with substance misusers

Generic workers with an occasional substance misuse portfolio	Generic workers with a substance misuse portfolio	Specialist workers
Nurse	Mental health nurse	Addiction nurses
Hospital pharmacist	Ambulance staff	Alcohol and drug worker
Teacher/lecturer	Connexions worker	Young people's substance
Early years worker	Youth worker	misuse worker
Citizens' Advice Bureau	Pupil Referral Unit	Drugs and employment
worker	teacher	coordinator
Social worker	Housing officer	Drugs unit police officer
Prison visitor	Care Leavers Team	Custody suite-based drug
Magistrate	social worker	worker
HM Customs worker	Homelessness worker	Progress2work advisor
Solicitor	Probation officer	Substance misuse
	Prison officer	commissioner
	Psychologist	Drug Action Team coordinator
	Community support	CARAT (counselling,
	officer	assessment, referral, advice
		and throughcare) worker
		Education drug advisor

Source: Home Office (2005) *Work Force Briefing, Tackling Drugs Changing Lives. Recruitment guidance for employers*. Home Office, London.

Examples of the types of role that might fall within each category are presented in Table 1.1.

The role of the nurse

In relation to substance misuse, nurses must assume a multitude of roles that focus on the provision of effective care, prevention and education (Rassool 1993). Such roles have been discussed in a document from the World Health Organization/ International Council of Nurses (WHO/ICN 1991) and are: provider of care, counsellor/therapist, educator/resource, advocate, health promoter, researcher, supervisor/leader and consultant. A brief description of the roles is shown in Table 1.2.

Nurses are uniquely positioned to enhance prevention and intervention strategies. For example, nurses have the opportunity and competence to assess smoking status, advise on the ill health effects of smoking, and assist in smoking cessation. The International Council of Nurses urges nurses around the world to be in the forefront of tobacco control. Nurses should develop partnerships with a broad range of other professional groups, women's and youth associations, the media, schools, government, and others committed to the prevention of substance misuse

Table 1.2 Nursing roles in relation to substance misuse.

Nursing role	Responsibilities
Provider of care	Caring for those who misuse or are affected by psychoactive substances
Counsellor/therapist	Focusing on the needs of individuals, their families and colleagues
Educator/resource	Providing health information to community groups, schools, families, individuals and to professional and non-professional groups
Advocate	Lobbying for change and improved care
Health promoter	Campaigning for policy and legislation to reduce demand for abused drugs
Researcher	Determining the most effective method of helping, caring and preventing substance misuse
Supervisor/leader	Guiding professionals and non-professionals
Consultant	Providing consultancy to professionals in this speciality

Source: WHO/ICN (World Health Organization/International Council of Nurses) (1991) *Roles of the Nurse in Relation to Substance Misuse*. ICN, Geneva. Reproduced with kind permission of the World Health Organization.

and reducing the harm resulting from the consequences of alcohol and drug misuse.

Hospital-based nurses

Patients who misuse psychoactive substances may be admitted to a variety of hospital-based settings and their health problems may or may not be related to alcohol and drug misuse. Patients attending hospital with alcohol-related problems fall into two broad categories: (i) those with a less severe drinking problem who may be amenable to brief interventions; and (ii) patients with features of alcohol dependence, requiring detoxification and ongoing treatment (Owens *et al.* 2005). The ranges of medical, surgical and psychiatric problems nurses are likely to encounter and their intervention strategies are shown in Table 1.3.

It is reported that up to 30% of male admissions and 15% of female admissions to general surgical and medical wards have alcohol-related problems (UK Alcohol Forum 1997). One in six people attending accident and emergency (A&E) departments for treatment have alcohol-related injuries or problems, rising to eight out of ten at peak times (HEA 1998), and one in seven acute hospital admissions are misusing alcohol (Canning 1999). For many drug misusers, A&E departments may be the first or only point of contact with health services, most often because of accidental overdoses and other crises (Gossop *et al.* 1995).

There has been a marked increase in the number of patients attending A&E departments following binge drinking and drug misuse. An increase of overnight alcohol-related emergencies to A&E after the introduction of new UK alcohol licensing legislation has also been reported (Newton *et al.* 2007). It is estimated

Table 1.3 Addiction problems encountered by hospital-based nurses.

Nurses	Problems	Interventions
Medical units	Unexplained fever. Acute or chronic infections of skins and joints. Unexplained cardiac murmurs. Endocarditis. Venous and arterial thrombosis. Jaundice. Abnormal liver function. Lymphadenopathy features of immunosuppression. Munchausen syndrome	Provision of total care. Screening. Taking a drug and alcohol history. Dealing with withdrawal symptoms and withdrawal. Harm reduction
Surgical units	Abscess. Acute abdominal pain. Intestinal obstruction (body packers). Vascular problems. Trauma (such as road traffic accidents or burns). Rhinitis. Rhinorrhoea	
Psychiatric nurse	Drug-induced psychosis (stimulants and alcohol). Drug-withdrawal psychosis (hypno-sedatives). Alcohol psychosis. Suicidal behaviour and depression as a result of substance misuse. Withdrawal symptoms. Dual diagnosis	Assessment of substance misuse and high-risk behaviours. Brief interventions. Cognitive therapy. Relapse prevention. Harm reduction
Accident and emergency nurse	Complications of substance misuse. Accidental overdoses. Intoxication. Withdrawal. Self-harm. Primary psychiatric symptoms	Brief assessment. Brief interventions. Dealing with self-harm. Management of overdose and withdrawal
Prison health care nurse	Alcohol and drug addiction. Self-harm. Dual diagnosis. HIV/AIDS and injecting drug use	Assessment of substance misuse and high-risk behaviours. Management of withdrawal. Harm reduction
Obstetric nurse/ midwife	Pregnant substance misusers	Harm reduction. Screening for cervical cytology. Smoking cessation. Maternal health, antenatal screening (hepatitis C, B and HIV), antenatal counselling, antenatal care and aftercare

that up to 5% of patients attending A&E departments present with primary psychiatric problems, whilst another 20–30% have psychiatric symptoms in addition to physical disorders (Ramirez & House 1997). The most common presenting psychiatric problem in most A&E departments is self-harm, typically constituting one-third of the total.

Table 1.4 Key points in reducing drug-related deaths.

Responses/Interventions	Needs/Problems
Injectors should be given injecting equipment	If needle exchange services are closed and they need injecting equipment
Encourage drug users to seek treatment	Reduce overdose and blood-borne infections
Hepatitis B immunisation for injectors who attend A&E	Should be a routine procedure
Risk of overdose due to loss of tolerance	Loss of tolerance after detoxification, rehabilitation or prison. Homeless injectors are a high-risk group
Long-term users and poly-drug users are at high risk of overdose	The more they overdose, the greater the risk of one of the overdoses being fatal
Provision of health information literature	Overdose prevention Viral transmission Local drug or alcohol services
Linking with local drug or alcohol agencies	Establish relationship with substance misuse services
Encourage drug or alcohol users to attend A&E	Non-judgmental and non-hostile attitude would be a positive experience for substance misusers and their friends or families

Source: adapted from NTA (National Treatment Agency) (2004) *Reducing Drug-related Deaths. Guidance for drug treatment providers*. NTA Publications, London.

The 'Models of Care' (NTA 2002) recommend that staff at A&E departments should include interventions strategies such as screening, provision of drug-related information and advice and referral to specialised alcohol or drug agencies. The key points of reducing drug-related deaths by A&E staff are presented in Table 1.4.

During the past decade, there has been a significant increase in the number of dedicated alcohol nurse specialists in hospitals (Owens *et al.* 2005). Alcohol nurse specialists have a multidimensional role ranging from providing advice on detoxification, screening for alcohol-related problems and optimising medical management through to providing ongoing support and information for referral for specialist alcohol treatment (Hillman *et al.* 2001).

Substance misuse is common among people with mental health problems and such dual needs should be met by mainstream services with the support of specialist advice (Department of Health 2002). Problems associated with alcohol/drug use are more common in mental health services, particularly in acute admission services. Mental health nurses in all settings should be able to respond to the needs of people with mental health and substance misuse problems (Department of Health 2006).

Prison health care services deal with the health needs of the prison population through the provision of general medical services and psychiatric treatment. Prison populations have a high concentration of people with a history of drug misuse: over one-third of the people received into British prisons each year are treated for opiate dependence (Home Office 2003).

Midwives provide support to women, their babies, their partners and families, from conception to the first phase of post-natal care. It is acknowledged that for some women this may be their only contact with the statutory health services. Late booking for antenatal care by women with problem drug and/or alcohol use is variously attributed either to lack of awareness of pregnancy, due to the menstrual disturbances and amenorrhoea that are common features of drug use, or else simply to lack of motivation (Hepburn 2004). Midwives can play an important role in nudging women who are misusing substances to make a positive change to substance-misusing behaviour. Another aspect of intervention includes the observation of babies undergoing withdrawal symptoms if they were born with a high degree of dependence on opiates.

Community-based nurses

A summary of the problems encountered by community-based nurses and their intervention strategies is presented in Table 1.5.

With the new NHS system focusing on identifying the needs for local services and on primary prevention with health improvement programmes, practice nurses are ideally placed to screen for drug misuse and for those with at-risk alcohol consumption, to deliver health information and brief interventions. There is some evidence suggesting that 13% of men and 2.5% of women having an alcohol use disorder consult their general practice (McMenamin 1997). In a study by Owens *et al.* (2000), the findings showed that practice nurses are happy to give advice regarding sensible drinking and routinely and appropriately take a history of alcohol intake, usually within well-woman and well-man clinics.

Community mental health nurses are exposed to a wide range of clients with varying degrees of psychiatric disorders and substance misuse. Community drug and alcohol teams may include community psychiatric nurses. Their work may cover the recognition of substance misusers, liaison with primary health care workers, for example general practitioners, in detoxification, motivation and relapse prevention, counselling, alcohol, drug and HIV (human immunodeficiency virus) education, and other harm minimisation work (Royal College of Psychiatrists 1997).

The use of tobacco, alcohol and illicit drugs by young people and school children is the source of much public concern. It is estimated that between 780 000 and 1.3 million children are affected by parental alcohol problems (Prime Minister's Strategy Unit 2004). School nurses are often asked to play a role in delivering health education/promotion (drug and sex education) under the personal, social and health education (PHSE) curriculum. A toolkit for school nurses has been developed to provide information about the effects of parental alcohol misuse on children and what can be done to support these children, both individually and within the wider school context (Alcohol Concern 2006).

Table 1.5 Addiction problems encountered by community-based nurses.

Nurse	Problems	Interventions
Community psychiatric nurse	Dual diagnosis problems related to withdrawal from alcohol or benzodiazepines, or opiates, blood-borne infections, amphetamine or cocaine psychosis	Assessment of mental health/ substance misuse problems. Counselling. Harm reduction. Relapse prevention. Cognitive therapy. Health education. Alternative therapies. Drug prescribing. Home detoxification. Prevention of substance misuse
Nurses in sexual health	HIV status. Sexually transmitted infections	Taking a drug and alcohol history. Pre- and post-test counselling. General counselling. Harm reduction
Practice nurse	General health problems. Wellness programme	Screening. Brief interventions. Provision of health information. Harm reduction. Smoking cessation clinic
District nurse	Different stages of illness	Early identification. Generic assessment. Health information. Harm reduction. Referral
School nurse	General health care of school children	Health education (drug and sex education). Health counselling. Referral to specialist and non-specialist agencies. Dealing with parental alcohol/ drug misuse
Occupational health nurse	General health care of workers	Health education. Screening for drugs and alcohol. Controlled drinking. Smoking cessation clinic. Harm reduction. Referral
Primary care mental health worker	Mental health needs	Brief interventions. Health information. Assessment and screening. Cognitive- behavioural therapies. Harm reduction

District nurses usually encounter patients at different stages in their illness and are responsible for the provision of total nursing care. They too have a role to play in prevention and harm reduction in relation to substance misuse.

The misuse of psychoactive substances in the workplace is one of the major concerns of management, professional organisations and occupational health staff. There is evidence to suggest that a policy on tobacco smoking or alcohol use can lead to reduced absenteeism, improved safety performances, lower maintenance costs, lower air-conditioning and ventilation costs, increased productivity, improve morale among non-smokers, fewer accidents and a lowered risk of losing skilled employees through premature retirement or death (McEwen 1991).

Primary care mental health workers provide additional, specialist services in primary care settings for people with mental health needs. One of the key functions is to help facilitate the transition towards primary care becoming the major arena of community mental health care and to facilitate the supply of basic therapeutic interventions such as cognitive behavioural therapies.

Substance misusers may come into contact with genitourinary medicine services as a result of concerns relating to their HIV status or sexually transmitted infections. Nurses working in sexual health need to have close working relationships with substance misuse and general services. Areas of intervention include taking a drug and alcohol history, sexual history, pre- and post-test counselling, general counselling, health education and harm reduction.

Addiction nurses: specialist alcohol and drug workers

Alcohol and drug workers or substance misuse workers come from a variety of professional backgrounds, including nursing, social work and the criminal justice system, and are found in statutory services, statutory and voluntary agencies and the private sector. They are regarded as drug and alcohol specialists. Nurses working in specialist alcohol and drug services have been ascribed occupational labels such as alcohol nurse, drug dependency nurse, chemical substance nurse, specialist nurse in addiction, and community psychiatric nurse (addiction) (Rassool 1997). It was not until the mid-1980s that addiction nursing as a clinical speciality, within the broader framework of mental health nursing, began to put down its clinical and academic roots.

The concept of addiction nursing was introduced in the literature in the UK by Rassool (1996). It is defined as a specialist branch of mental health nursing concerned with treatment interventions aimed at those individuals whose health problems are directly related to the use and misuse of psychoactive substances and to other addictive behaviours such as eating disorders and gambling (Rassool 1997). The scope of professional practice in addiction nursing incorporates the activities of clinical practice, education, policy making, research and an expanded role in the prescribing of drugs (Rassool 2004).

Addiction nurses practice in a variety of settings including smoking cessation clinics, mobile methadone clinics, outreach work with drug-using commercial sex workers, and satellite clinics for homeless drinkers; they are also involved in the development of multiprofessional post-graduate educational programmes in addictive behavior (Rassool 2000). Addiction nurses provide a range of physical and psychosocial interventions in the management and comprehensive treatment of substance misusers. The interventions include total nursing care, management of withdrawal and detoxification, prescribing, support, advice and basic counselling, harm reduction, family therapy and cognitive behavioural therapies such as relapse prevention. They also have a key worker role in the shared care approach, perform risk assessment and act as an advocate. Some nurses practice in a 'social work model' and can address family and personal relationships, child care, housing, income support and criminal justice issues (Department of Health 1999a).

Confidentiality

Under statutory law and professional codes of practice, nurses, midwives and allied professionals have a professional duty of care relating to respecting and maintaining patient confidentiality. The professional ethical obligations for nurses are set out in the Nursing and Midwifery Council's *Code of Professional Practice* (NMC 2002). It is stated that:

> To trust another person with private and personal information about yourself is a significant matter. If the person to whom that information is given is a nurse, midwife or health visitor, the patient or client has a right to believe that this information, given in confidence, will only be used for the purposes for which it was given and will not be released to others without their permission. The death of a patient or client does not give you the right to break confidentiality.

Nurses, whether working in the NHS or the private sector, should also observe any government guidelines on confidentiality such as the Department of Health's (2003) code of practice on confidentiality. Information provided in confidence should not be used or disclosed in a form that might identify a patient without his or her consent (Department of Health 2007). The person's right to confidentiality means that all clients must have this clearly defined and explained to them before being asked to reveal any personal information. Information can be provided to third parties on their behalf *only* if their specific written permission is provided before this occurs. Informed consent is an ongoing agreement by a person to receive treatment and undergo procedures (or participate in research), after the risks, benefits and alternatives have been adequately explained to them (Royal College of Nursing 2005). The consent should be documented, accessible in the client's notes and subject to regular review. For more comprehensive information see *Patient Confidentiality* (Department of Health 2007) and *Guidance for Access to Health Records* (Department of Health 2003).

Record keeping: case notes and electronic care records

The keeping of records of patients as part of a care plan is a basic requirement of health and social care practice. A record is 'anything that contains information (in any media) which has been created or gathered as a result of any aspect of the work of NHS employees' (Department of Health 1999b). Within the Data Protection Act 1998, a health record is defined as a record consisting of information about the physical or mental health or condition of an identifiable individual made by or on behalf of a health professional in connection with the care of that individual. The Data Protection Act 1998 gives every living person or their authorized representative the right to apply for access to their health records irrespective of when they were compiled. The process of keeping records involves consideration by third parties, including courts of law and other health or social care professionals. Nurses should keep records that are simple, accurate, legible and up-to-date. Clinical records must be kept confidential at all times and stored in a secure place.

Under the NHS Electronic Care Records system, everyone will have a computer-based care file with basic information to provide health care staff with quicker access to reliable information. The NHS Care Records Service aims to make caring across organisational boundaries safer and more efficient. This will mean that instead of having separate records in all the different services, key workers will have access to the information they need. The electronic patient records are available to staff whenever a client visits hospital or community-based services. Access to the electronic record is strictly password controlled to maintain patient confidentiality at all times.

Summary of key points

- Nurses are usually the first point of contact for patients who have potential or early alcohol and drug problems.
- The extent and nature of the substantial health and social problems associated with substance misuse highlight the pressing need for nurses to respond to the needs of substance misusers.
- Roles in the substance misuse field are characterised by the level and frequency of contact with substance misuse and substance misusers.
- The exchange and sharing of information has to be done whilst observing the code of practice regarding confidentiality and should be underpinned by clear policies and procedures.
- Record keeping is a basic health and social care practice and is applicable to all services.

References

Alcohol Concern (2006) *Toolkit for School Nurses*. Alcohol Concern, London: http://www.alcoholandfamilies.org.uk/documents/SN/sn-tools_index.htm.

Canning U.P., Kennell-Webb S.A., Marshall E.J., Wessely S.C. & Peters T.J. (1999) Substance misuse in acute general medical admissions. *Quarterly Journal of Medicine*, 92(6), 319–326.

Department of Health (1999a) *Drug Misuse and Dependence. Guidelines on clinical management*. Department of Health, London.

Department of Health (1999b) *For the Record: managing records in NHS Trusts and Health Authorities*. HSC 1999/053. Department of Health, London: www.doh.gov.uk/nhsexec/manrec.htm (accessed 10 June 2009).

Department of Health (2002) *Mental Health Policy Implementation Guide: dual diagnosis good practice guide*. Department of Health, London: www.dh.gov.uk/PublicationsAndStatistics/Publications/PublicationsPolicyAndGuidance/PublicationsPolicyAndGuidanceArticle/fs/en?CONTENT_ID=4009058&chk=sCQrQr.

Department of Health (2003) *Guidance for Access to Health Records*. Department of Health, London: www.doh.gov.uk.

Department of Health (2006) *From Values to Action: the Chief Nursing Officer's review of mental health nursing*. Department of Health, London.

Department of Health (2007) *Patient Confidentiality*. Department of Health, London: www.doh.gov.uk.

Gossop M., Marsden, J., Edwards C., Wilson A., Segar G., Stewart D. & Lehmann P. (1995) *The October Report. The National Treatment Outcome Research Study: a report prepared for the Task Force*. Department of Health, London.

HEA (Health Education Authority) (1998) Perceptions of alcohol related attendances in A&E departments in England: a national survey. *Alcohol and Alcoholism*, 33(4), 354–361.

Hillman A., McCann B. & Walker N. P. (2001) Specialist alcohol liaison services in general hospitals improve engagement in alcohol rehabilitation and treatment outcome. *Health Bulletin*, 59(6), 420–423.

Hepburn M. (2004) Substance abuse in pregnancy. *Current Obstetrics and Gynaecology*, 14, 419–425.

Home Office (2003a) *An Analysis of CARAT Research Data as at 3 December 2002*, Research, Development and Statistics Directorate, London: Home Office.

Home Office (2005) *Work Force Briefing, Tackling Drugs Changing Lives. Recruitment guidance for employers*. Home Office, London: www. homeoffice.gov.uk/publication-search/drugstrategy/WorkforceBriefing-Jobs?view=Binary.

McEwen J. (1991) Interventions in the workplace. In I. Glass (ed.) *The International Handbook of Addiction Behaviour*, pp. 307–312. Routledge, London.

McMenamin J.P. (1997) Detecting young adults with alcohol use disorder in a general practice. *New Zealand Medical Journal*, 110, 127–128.

Newton A., Sarker S.J., Pahal G.S., van den Bergh E. & Young C. (2007) Impact of the new UK licensing law on emergency hospital attendances: a cohort study. *Emergency Medicine Journal*, 24(8), 532–534.

NMC (Nursing and Midwifery Council) (2002) *The Code of Professional Conduct*. NMC, London.

NMC (Nursing and Midwifery Council) (2007) *The Code: standards of conduct, performance and ethics for nurses and midwives*. NMC, London. http://www.nmc-uk.org/aDisplayDocument.aspx?documentID=5982.

NTA (National Treatment Agency) (2002) *Models of Care for Treatment of Adult Drug Misuers. Parts 1 and 2*. NTA Publications, London.

NTA (National Treatment Agency) (2004) *Reducing Drug-related Deaths. Guidance for drug treatment providers*. NTA Publications, London: http://www.nta.nhs.uk/publications/documents/nta_guidance__for__drug__treatment__providers_drdpro.pdf.

Owens L., Gilmore I.T. & Pirmohamed M. (2000) General practice nurses' knowledge of alcohol use and misuse: a questionnaire survey. *Alcohol and Alcoholism*. 35(3), 259–262.

Owens L., Gilmore I.T. & Pirmohamed M. (2005) How do the NHS general hospitals in England deal with patients with alcohol-related problems? A questionnaire survey. *Alcohol and Alcoholism*, 40(5), 409–412.

Prime Minister's Strategy Unit (2004) *Alcohol Harm Reduction Strategy for England*. Cabinet Office, London: http://www.cabinetoffice.gov.uk/strategy/work_areas/alcohol_misuse.aspx.

Ramirez A. & House A. (1997) ABC of mental health: common mental health problems in the general hospital. *British Medical Journal*, 314, 1679–1681.

Rassool G.H. (1993) Nursing and substance misuse: responding to the challenge. *Journal of Advanced Nursing*, 18(9), 1401–1407.

Rassool G.H. (1996) Addiction nursing and substance misuse: a slow response to partial accommodation. *Journal of Advanced Nursing*, 24(2), 425–427.

Rassool G.H. (1997) Addiction nursing – towards a new paradigm: the UK experience. In G.H. Rassool & M. Gafoor (eds) *Addiction Nursing – perspectives on professional and clinical practice*. Nelson Thornes, Cheltenham, UK.

Rassool G.H. (2000) Addiction: global problem and global response complacency or commitment? *Journal of Advanced Nursing*, 32(3), 505–508.

Rassool G.H. (2004) Prescription for change: perspectives on prescribing authority for addiction nurses in the United Kingdom. *Journal of Addictions Nursing*, 15(4), 193–197.

Rassool G.H. (2009) *Alcohol and Drug Misuse. A handbook for student and health professionals*. Routledge, Oxford.

Rassool G.H. & Oyefeso N. (1993) The need for substance misuse education in health studies curriculum: a case for nursing education. *Nurse Education Today*, 13, 107–110.

Royal College of Psychiatrists (1997) *Community Psychiatric Nursing*. Occasional Paper No. OP40. Royal College of Psychiatrists, London.

Royal College of Nursing (2005) *Informed Consent in Health and Social Care Research*. Royal College of Nursing, London.

UK Alcohol Forum (1997) *Guidelines for the Management of Alcohol Problems in Primary Care and General Psychiatry*. Tangent Medical Education, London.

WHO/ICN (World Health Organization/International Council of Nurses) (1991) *Roles of the Nurse in Relation to Substance Misuse*. ICN, Geneva.

2 Myths, Attitudes and Confidence Skills in Addiction

Our understanding of addiction is based on a lay foundation as much as on our scientific understanding of addiction, which is relatively new. Our understanding of alcohol and drug addiction is embedded in belief systems and attitudes. We have developed a number of myths about addiction and these have been made legitimate. We will need to dispel some of the most popular myths as evidence suggests that they are false. The myths have a significant influence in our understanding of addiction and our interaction with alcohol and drug users and misusers. Many factors impact on nurses and other health care professionals' willingness to intervene with individuals who use drugs and alcohol. These factors include knowledge, training, organisational structure and policies, and previous positive or negative experiences (Rassool 2009). Interactions with alcohol and drug users and misusers are also tied up with our myths, attitudes and confidence.

In this chapter, there are a number of self-assessed activities to examine the myths of addiction, our personal use of alcohol and drugs, attitudes towards substance misusers and intervention confidence skills in working with substance misusers. In order to understand the nature and reasons behind the use of alcohol and drugs, you will need first to understand your own 'dependence'. You need also to be more aware of your own attitude towards substance misusers. Understanding why an individual becomes dependent on alcohol or drug may enable you to have a more positive attitude (feeling, thinking and behaviour) about substance misusers and facilitate them to change their behaviour.

Myths about alcohol and drugs

In Activity 2.1, you will need to consider whether the statements are fact or fiction. It would be worthwhile to look for evidence to support the statements. The answers appear at the end of this chapter.

Activity 2.1 Please tick the appropriate box to state whether the statement is fact or fiction

	Statement	Fact	Fiction
1	There are no degrees of addiction		
2	Alcohol or drug addiction is an intentional behaviour		
3	Individuals who use drugs on a regular basis will become dependent or addicted		
4	Individuals who continue to misuse alcohol or drugs after treatment are failures		
5	Individuals need to reach rock bottom before they can get any help		
6	Users of drugs or alcohol have defect characters and are bad		
7	The number of individuals relapsing shows that treatment is not effective		
8	Addiction ends after detoxification and the withdrawal syndrome is gone		
9	Babies born of mothers who use drugs during pregnancy are born 'addicted'		
10	All drugs damage brain cells		
11	Addicts can stop using drugs/drinking by just attending Alcoholics or Narcotics Anonymous		
12	There is an 'addictive personality'		
13	Individuals that become alcoholics or problem drug users have mental issues that lead them to addiction		
14	Recovering alcoholics can drink socially		
15	I can smoke one cigarette and maintain my quit programme		

Personal use of psychoactive substances

In this section, you will consider your own use of alcohol and drugs. Self-awareness of one's own drug (legal, prescribed or illicit) or alcohol use should enable you to be more cognisant about the nature and reasons behind the misuse of alcohol and drugs. This activity is based on the 'addiction' of substances (alcohol and drugs), things, people or activities (Scottish Drugs Training Project, University of Stirling). For example, people may be dependent on alcohol, coffee, tea, chocolate, a first cigarette on waking up, jogging, horse racing, the internet or soap operas; abstinence from the substances, activities or things would create an emptiness in your daily routine. Please undertake Activity 2.2.

The reasons why people use drugs and continue to use drugs are two different propositions. The reasons may or may not be the same. Physical and psychological withdrawals of psychoactive substances are discussed in Chapters 6–12.

Activity 2.2   Personal use of addictive substances/activities/people/things

---

1 List your dependence/dependencies:
  (a) Substances:
  (b) Activities:
  (c) People/things:
2 (a) What are the reasons you think you may be dependent?
  (b) Why do you need them?
  (c) What do they do for you?
3 (a) How would you feel if you had to give up your preferred choice of dependence?
  (b) Would it be easy or difficult?
  (c) Would you have physical or psychological withdrawal symptoms or both?

Source: Scottish Drugs Training Project, University of Stirling.

Attitudes and stigmatisation

An attitude is the way we feel, think or behave towards an individual or thing. For example, nurses can have a positive or negative attitude towards working with alcohol and drug misusers. That is, they may be reluctant to work with substance misusers because they perceive alcohol and drug misusers as unpleasant and over-demanding. Attitudes are influenced by a variety of factors, including past experiences (positive and negative), knowledge, education, context of the situation, and cultural and religious factors. Changing an attitude is a complex problem as an individual's attitudes may be closely tied to their personal values, belief system or important aspects of their self-identity (Wood 1998). Attitudes towards substance misusers represent one factor within this wider set that may impact on health professionals' responses. In this context, attitudes towards alcohol and drug misusers can be broadly categorised as professional or personal views. Professional attitudes refer to beliefs concerning professional practice such as role legitimacy (e.g. is it appropriate for me to respond to alcohol use within my professional role?), confidence (perceived level of skills and abilities) and perceived efficacy of available treatments and interventions (Rassool 2009). Personal attitudes refer to feelings and beliefs that stem from the stigmatised nature of drug use, for example blame and anger.

Attitudes of health care professionals towards substance misusers exert a significant influence on their readiness to intervene and the quality of such interventions. Negative attitudes have been associated with the reluctance of substance misusers to utilise the health services, reduced likelihood to pursue referrals and the reluctance of health care professionals to engage in management and treatment with substance abusers (McLaughlin *et al.* 2000; Mistral & Velleman 2001).

Complete Activity 2.3 and reflect about your attitudes towards alcohol and drug misusers. Write in your reflective journal about your own substance use and your attitude towards substance misusers.

Activity 2.3 Rassool Attitude Towards Substance Misusers Questionnaire (RATSMQ-10)

The statements below reflect several different opinions, beliefs and viewpoints about substance use and misuse. Please indicate how strongly you agree or disagree with each statement. To complete the instrument please place a tick in the box that best reflects how strongly you agree or disagree with each statement.

1 Personal use of illicit drugs should be legal in the confines of one's home.

Strongly agree	Agree	Uncertain	Disagree	Strongly Disagree

2 Drug addicts suffer from feelings of inferiority.

Strongly agree	Agree	Uncertain	Disagree	Strongly Disagree

3 People who use illicit drugs do not respect authority.

Strongly agree	Agree	Uncertain	Disagree	Strongly Disagree

4 Heroin is so addictive that no one can really recover once he or she becomes an addict.

Strongly agree	Agree	Uncertain	Disagree	Strongly Disagree

5 Rehabilitation of drug misusers always fails.

Strongly agree	Agree	Uncertain	Disagree	Strongly Disagree

6 Illicit drug users are a monetary and social drain on the community.

Strongly agree	Agree	Uncertain	Disagree	Strongly Disagree

7 Compulsory treatment is necessary for those who are addicted to drugs and/or alcohol.

Strongly agree	Agree	Uncertain	Disagree	Strongly Disagree

8 Alcohol misusers should be referred to a specialist once health problems are identified.

Strongly agree	Agree	Uncertain	Disagree	Strongly Disagree

9 Those who are addicted to drugs are unpleasant to work with.

Strongly agree	Agree	Uncertain	Disagree	Strongly Disagree

10 Drug addicts are stigmatised by health care professionals.

Strongly agree	Agree	Uncertain	Disagree	Strongly Disagree

Rassool Attitude Towards Substance Misusers Questionnaire, © G. Hussein Rassool 2004. Permission should be obtained from the author for use of the questionnaire beyond personal use.

Activity 2.4   Addiction Intervention Skills Questionnaire

To complete the instrument, please place a tick in the box that best reflects your confidence level.

	Low confidence	Moderate confidence	High confidence
Providing alcohol use education and prevention information			
Recognising signs and symptoms of alcohol problems			
Talking to patients about the risks of alcohol misuse			
Taking an alcohol history			
Referring patients for alcohol treatment			
Providing care for patients with alcohol problems			
Providing drug use education and prevention information			
Recognising signs and symptoms of drug problems			
Talking to patients about the risks of drug misuse			
Taking a drug history			
Referring patients to drug treatment			
Providing care for patients with drug problems			
Giving health risk information on prescribed medication			
Informing smokers about the health risks of tobacco smoking			
Providing tobacco education and prevention information			
Knowledge of drug and alcohol services			

Addiction Intervention Skills Questionnaire, © G. Hussein Rassool 2004. Permission should be obtained from the author for use of the questionnaire beyond personal use.

Intervention confidence skills

If you have a belief in yourself and in your competences or abilities in providing optimal care to any group of patients, you will have the readiness to work with alcohol and drug misusers. In addition, having a positive attitude or therapeutic optimism will influence your interventions with substance misusers. Nurses will have some areas of their nursing or health activities where they feel quite confident, while at the same time they may not feel at all confident in other areas. By taking a positive attitude this may enable the development of confidence skills in working with alcohol and drug misusers. Please complete the Questionnaire of Intervention Confidence Skills in working with substance misusers (Activity 2.4).

When you have completed the book or a course, you should return and complete this questionnaire for a second time. It would be valuable for you to compare the two sets of answers in relation to your intervention confidence skills.

Summary of key points

- Our understanding of addiction is based on a lay foundation and scientific understanding.
- Our understanding of alcohol and drug addiction is rooted in myths, belief systems and attitudes.
- There is a need to be self-aware about own dependence on substances, things, activities or people.
- Reflect on your own attitude towards those with alcohol and drug problems.
- It is important to develop a positive attitude in order to enhance the quality of care given to those with alcohol or drug problems.
- By taking a positive attitude this may enable the development of confidence skills in working with alcohol and drug misusers.

Statements and responses to Activity 2.1

1 *Myth*: There are no degrees of addiction

Fact: The progression of an addiction reflects a broad spectrum, ranging from no use to dependence. At one extreme, there is no use of alcohol or other drugs. An experimental user may misuse a psychoactive substances on a few occasions. Then there is the occasional or recreational user who functions at a normal level at home and is in employment. There are usually no adverse medical or social consequences as a result of recreational use, as in the case of controlled drinking. At the other extreme, the dependent user has progressed to regular and problematic use of a psychoactive drug or has become a poly-drug user. There is a formal system for measuring the severity of a patient's addiction: the ASI (Addiction Severity Index).

2 *Myth*: Alcohol or drug addiction is an intentional behaviour

Fact: The choice to try a psychoactive substance for the first time may be a voluntary decision. But as times passes, however, even this choice may be influenced by such factors as peer pressure, self-esteem and availability or accessibility. Biological conditions may also predispose an individual to craving that may result in compulsive and even chaotic drug use. In this state, the freedom of choice diminishes and usually disappears.

3 *Myth*: Individuals who use drugs on a regular basis will become dependent or addicted

Fact: Not all individuals who use drugs or alcohol on a regular basis will become dependent. Research shows that the risk for developing alcohol or drug addiction does indeed run in families. Genetic and other psychosocial factors may also increase the risk of addiction and dependence. Some individuals will get addicted and others may not, for example users who take drug or alcohol on a recreational, controlled basis.

4 *Myth*: Individuals who continue to misuse alcohol or drugs after treatment are failures

Fact: Addiction is a chronic disorder and occasional relapse does not mean failure. Completing a treatment package is merely the first step on the road to recovery and a drug-free lifestyle. The road to recovery is a long process and frequently requires multiple treatment attempts. Addicts are most vulnerable to drug use during the few months immediately following their release from treatment as psychosocial factors can easily trigger a relapse.

5 *Myth*: Individuals need to reach rock bottom before they can get any help

Fact: There is no evidence to suggest that individuals need to reach rock bottom before they can get any help. In fact, the earlier individuals get help, the more likely they are to improve their journey to the recovery process. However, pressure from family members, partners and employers, as well as insight to the fact that they have a problem, can be powerful motivating factors for individuals to seek treatment.

6 *Myth*: Users of drugs or alcohol have defect characters and are bad

Fact: There is no evidence to suggest that alcohol and drug misusers are 'bad' people with character flaws, but addiction to drugs may involve changes in mood, memory processes and behavioural skills.

7 *Myth*: The number of individuals relapsing shows that treatment is not effective

Fact: Relapses occurs not only with drug addiction but also with other disorders such as diabetes, cancer and hypertension. It is a fact that relapse is high but that does not mean that treatment is ineffective or not worthwhile. There is evidence to suggest that drug treatment reduces drug use by 40–60% and can significantly decrease criminal activity during and after treatment. In addition, there is also evidence that drug addiction treatment reduces the risk of HIV (human immunodeficiency virus) infection.

8 *Myth*: Addiction ends after detoxification and the withdrawal syndrome is gone

Fact: Detoxification is only one stage on the journey to recovery. Although at the end of the withdrawal process, pain caused by the body's dependence on the psychoactive substance is gone, the underlying psychosocial problems remain.

9 *Myth*: Babies born of mothers who use drugs during pregnancy are born 'addicted'

Fact: For addiction to occur, it requires a fully developed nervous system and the presence of the drug. First, not all babies are susceptible to addiction even if they are exposed to a drug. Second, when drug-exposed babies are seen to have withdrawal or other signs of distress at birth, people readily assume that the babies are 'addicted'.

10 *Myth*: All drugs damage brain cells

Fact: Relatively few psychoactive substances have been shown to damage brain cells through a toxic effect – those that do, for example, include alcohol (high doses over a long time), 'inhalants' (paint thinner, glue, correction fluids, hair sprays), methamphetamine and MDMA (3,4-methylenedioxymethamphetamine, commonly known as ecstasy) (shown in animal studies with high doses, but not yet in humans).

11 *Myth*: Addicts can stop using drugs/drinking by just attending Alcoholics or Narcotics Anonymous

Fact: Those attending a 12-step programme of Alcoholics or Narcotics Anonymous give a lifelong commitment. This approach to treatment does not suit all addicts. Some individuals require more intensive intervention strategies or structured environments.

12 *Myth*: There is an 'addictive personality'

Fact: Personality is a complex characteristic and the role of personality in addiction is uncertain. Certainly, there is little evidence for an addictive personality. However, there are a number of personality types that have been associated with addiction. The strongest evidence supports the 'antisocial personality'.

13 *Myth*: Individuals that become alcoholics or problem drug users have mental issues that lead them to addiction

Fact: This may be so in some cases, as the prevalence of disorders such as depression and bipolar disorder is high amongst problem drinkers. However, not everyone that is addicted to alcohol or drugs is suffering from a psychiatric disorder; this is a blanket statement and simply is not true.

14 *Myth*: Recovering alcoholics can drink socially

Fact: There are a few scientific studies that suggest that recovering alcoholics can drink socially.

15 *Myth*: I can smoke one cigarette and maintain my quit programme

Fact: For the vast majority of smokers, re-introducing nicotine after quitting leads back to full-time smoking. There is no such thing as just one cigarette for a nicotine addict.

References

McLaughlin D., McKenna H. & Leslie J.C. (2000) The perceptions and aspirations of illicit drug users hold towards health care staff and the care they receive. *Journal of Psychiatric and Mental Health Nursing*, 7, 435–441.

Mistral W. & Velleman R. (2001) Substance-misusing patients in primary care: incidence, services provided and problems. A survey of general practitioners in Wiltshire. *Drugs: Education, Prevention and Policy*, 8, 61–71.

Rassool G.H. (2009) *Alcohol and Drug Misuse. A handbook for student and health professionals*. Routledge, London.

Wood I. (1998) Effects of continuing professional education on the clinical practice of nurses: a review of the literature. *International Journal of Nursing Studies*, 35(3), 125–131.

3 Addiction and Society

Alcohol and drug misuse remains a global health problem despite efforts in the legislative control, prevention, intervention strategies, treatment and rehabilitation. We are all addicted to something whether it is alcohol or drugs, chocolate, texting on mobile phones, jogging or watching soap operas on TV. Most of us have some compulsive behaviour patterns, but most of the time these do not cause us any physical or psychological harm or both. The danger arises when we use a substance or thing in an uncontrolled, compulsive way despite the physical, psychological or social harm it causes. In most societies, many individuals will consume alcoholic beverages and others will use illicit psychoactive substances. Individuals have learned that using psychoactive substances makes them feel good. However, the consumption of alcohol or drugs may result in the development of dependence and addiction for a sizeable minority. The nature and extent of the problem will depend upon the individual, the type of psychoactive active substance(s) and the environment. The public health problem related to alcohol and drug misuse is not confined to illicit drugs but to prescriptions of painkillers and a new class of 'happy and magic pills' that doctors are prescribing.

Addiction for Nurses By G. Hussein Rassool. © 2010 G. Hussein Rassool

Historical perspective

The historical context of the use of psychoactive substances helps us to understand the distinctive nature of the use and misuse of alcohol and drugs in today's society. The records of ancient civilisations provide evidence of the use of alcohol and plants with psychoactive properties. Alcohol and drugs have been used for many centuries for medicinal, religious, cultural and recreational purposes and as a social lubricant. However, in the 1920s, Britain had its first notable drug panic. The detection of a drug underground of cocaine and heroin provided a way of speaking simultaneously about women, race, sex and the nation's place in the world. In addition, the remnants of this belief still remain in the public consciousness. In the past, the outlawing of drugs was the consequence not of their pharmacology but their association with social groups that were perceived as potentially dangerous (Kohn 1992).

Alcohol

The word 'alcohol' comes from the Arabic language, and may be derived from *al-kuhl*, the name of an early distilled substance. In ancient Egypt, alcohol was used for pleasure, nutrition, medicine, rituals, remuneration and funerary purposes. At the height of the Roman Empire, both ceremonial drinking (confined to banquets and special occasions) and casual drinking were common. Alcohol achieved dominance in European nations through the ritualisation of alcohol in Christian Europe and the revulsion of mind-altering psychoactive substances by the church (Gossop 1989). In England both ale and beer were at the top of lists of products given to lords for rent. Whitaker (1987) suggested that distilled alcohol inflicted more havoc on North American Indians and Australians Aborigines than any other drug throughout history.

Amphetamines

Amphetamines, synthesised in 1887, were marketed in the form of a benzedrine inhaler for use in the treatment of nasal congestion, mild depression, schizophrenia, alcoholism and obesity.

During the Second World War, the armed forces used amphetamines to function under stressful and physically demanding conditions. During the 1950s, there was over-prescription of amphetamines by doctors for use in the treatment of obesity and other common conditions. More recently, amphetamines have also been used in the treatment of narcolepsy and hyperactivity in children. It was not until the 1960s that amphetamine misuse erupted in the UK among young people and subsequently resulted in an epidemic of methamphetamine injection. The use of the stimulant is also widespread amongst athletes to enhance their performances.

Cannabis

Cannabis sativa (or Indian hemp), more commonly known as cannabis or mari-juana, was one of the first plants to be cultivated for its non-food properties, and was primarily harvested for its fibre. The drug was used for its pharmacological properties in the treatment of physical and psychological problems and for reli-gious functions. The exposure of cannabis in Europe was also influenced by printed literature and the medical profession began to show an interest in the use of cannabis by the middle of the nineteenth century. An Irish physician, William O'Shaughnessy, described the medical application of cannabis whilst in India and introduced it in Great Britain (Bloomquist 1971). In France, the use and effects of hashish were described by a small group of writers, intellectuals and artists; in the 1840s, Le Club des Hachishins (The Hashish Club) was founded in an exclu-sive hotel in Paris. Despite its attraction as a recreational or intoxicating drug, it did not immediately spread in Europe. However, the widespread use of cannabis or hashish for its psychoactive properties in Europe in the 1960s seems to have occurred as a result of the cultural movement of the young generation imported from the United States (Rassool 2009). The plant grows freely throughout the world but is indigenous to Central Asia and the Himalayan region and is grown in at least 172 countries, often in small plots by the users themselves (UNODC 2007). During the last four decades, cannabis has remained the most frequently used illicit drug in the UK.

Cocaine

The use of the coca leaf dates back to the Inca civilisations and their descendants and it was used for medicinal purposes, religious significance, and in rituals, burials and other special occasions. The Spanish conquistadores encouraged the Inca to use the coca leaf in the belief that it helped the Inca to work longer and harder. In fact, because of its social importance, the Spanish eventually took over coca production and distribution and used coca as a tool to control the conquered population (Petersen 1977). In the 1850s European chemists were able to isolate the far more potent ingredient in the leaf, which they called cocaine.

Freud recommended the use of cocaine as a local anaesthetic and as a treatment for drug addiction, alcoholism, depression, various neuroses, indigestion, asthma and syphilis. By the 1880s cocaine was widely available in patent medicines that could be obtained without prescription. These included Mariani's Coca Wine, a best-seller in Europe, and Coca-Cola. Cocaine became very popular and was also sold in cigarettes, in nose sprays and in chewing gum (Gossop 1989). It was not until the 1980s that cocaine became the 'rich man's' drug of choice and its accept-ance has been fostered by an association with glamorous images and compounded by the idea of the 'non-addictive' nature of the drug. Consumption of cocaine has increased significantly in Europe, doubling or tripling in several countries over the last decade (UNODC 2007).

Caffeine

Caffeine is the world's most popular psychoactive substance and was used medicinally and for religious purposes. During the seventeenth century, coffee drinking spread from the Arab world and Persia to Britain and other European countries. In eighteenth century England, coffee was seen as an alternative to sex and as a cure for alcohol intoxication. The drinking of coffee and the spread of coffee houses shocked public opinion at that time. According to Ghodse (1995: xi), attempts were made in different countries 'to close down the coffee houses which were seen as centres of sedition and dissent and to ban the use of coffee altogether'. Coffee is the major source of caffeine though other familiar psychoactive substances such as tea, cocoa and chocolate also contain caffeine.

Hallucinogenic drugs

Hallucinogenic drugs were originally called 'phantastica' (Lewin 1964) and during the 1960s the drugs were referred to as 'psychedelics' (Stevens 1987). They have played an important role in cultural and religious traditions and were used as part of religious rituals and practices and in the healing of the sick. It was the synthetic hallucinogens such as LSD (lysergic acid diethylamide) that came under scientific and medical scrutiny. Initially, LSD was primarily used as an adjunct to psychotherapy and later in the treatment of alcoholism, drug dependence, sexual problems and psychotic and neurotic disorders. By the early 1960s the drug was used by the emerging 'hippy' subculture for spiritual enlightenment and for mystical peak experiences. Throughout the 1980s in the UK there was a decline in the use of LSD but it resurfaced in the late 1980s together with other hallucinogens in the 'rave' subculture. Ecstasy (MDMA or 3,4-methylenedioxymethamphetamine), although not a new drug, appeared on the scene in 1985 and since then there has been an increase in the consumption of both ecstasy and LSD by young people. The drug was first used as an appetite suppressant.

Opium

Opium is an extract of the exudates derived from seed pods of the opium poppy. The opium plant produces lots of small black seeds called poppy seeds. Arab physicians such as Ibn-Sina (or Avicenna, 980–1037), used opium extensively, writing special treatises on its preparations and recommended the plant especially for diarrhoea and diseases of the eye. In England, opium was chiefly used as a narcotic and a hypnotic. Thomas Sydenham, the seventeenth century pioneer of English medicine, introduced the use of opium in medicine. In the nineteenth century, laudanum, a mixture of alcohol solution and tincture of opium, could be bought over the counter at any grocer's shop and for decade it was every family's favourite remedy for minor aches and pains (Royal College of Psychiatrists 1989). Other substances with opium-based preparations such as Godfrey's Cordial, a soothing syrup of opium tincture, were effective against colic; Street's Infants' Quietness, Atkinson's Infants' Preservative and Mrs. Winslow's Soothing Syrup were all used for babies and young children for sedation. In effect, opium was used in preference to alcohol and in various forms for endemic conditions such as malaria.

Morphine was first isolated from opium in 1805 by a German pharmacist, Wilhelm Sertürner and he named it morphium – after Morpheus, the Greek god of dreams. The development of the hypodermic syringe in the mid-nineteenth century allowed the injection of pure morphine. In the late nineteenth century, morphine became the drug of choice for high society and middle class profession-als. It was believed that injecting morphine was not addictive and would be effec-tive treating those with opium dependence. In 1874, English pharmacist C. R. Alder Wright boiled morphine and acetic acid to produce diacetylmorphine. Diacetylmorphine was synthesised and marketed commercially by the German pharmaceutical giant, Bayer. In 1898, Bayer launched the best-selling drug brand of all time, Heroin (http://opioids.com/.)

Tobacco

Tobacco is a plant that grows natively in North and South America. It is in the same family as the potato, pepper and poisonous nightshade. Tobacco was believed to be a cure-all, and was used to dress wounds, as well as a painkiller for toothache. In South and Central America, a complex system of religious and political rites was developed around tobacco use (Imperial Tobacco Canada 2007). In 1632, it was illegal to smoke publicly in Massachusetts, America – a reflection of the moral belief prevailing at this period amongst the new settlers in America. The same policy is nowadays applied in many countries to promote public health.

In 1847, the famous British firm Philip Morris was established, selling hand-rolled Turkish cigarettes. During the Crimean War (1854–1856) and the two world wars, soldiers were offered cigarettes to overcome the misery of food deprivation or they were included in a soldier's rations. During the 1950s, important epide-miological studies provided the first powerful links between smoking and lung cancer. But it was not until 1971 that tobacco manufacturers in the UK voluntarily put health warnings on cigarette packs. During the 1980s and 1990s, the tobacco industry started marketing heavily in developing countries in Asia and Africa. In recent years, there is growing evidence that the tobacco industry knew all along that cigarettes are harmful, but continued to market and sell them. During the late 1990s smoking became prohibited in bars and restaurants in many countries and subsequently this has been followed by a total ban in public places.

Different cultures and alcohol and drug use

Alcohol and drugs have been the most commonly used intoxicating psychoactive substances in almost all cultures for centuries. However, the nature and extent of substance misuse vary widely among different ethno-cultural communities (Johnson & Carroll 1995). In many countries in the northern hemispheres, alcohol use is widely accepted as a social lubricant for promoting relaxation and sociability. In abstinence-based cultures, especially in Islamic countries, alcohol use is strictly prohibited under any circumstances. In many cultures young people are introduced to alcohol early in life as a normal part of daily living. In some cultures, other psychoactive substances are given as part of the rites of passage for young people. Some ethnic communities, including Chinese, Japanese and Korean, have a deficiency or absence of the liver enzyme, alcohol dehydrogenase (ALDH). The intake of alcohol may result in vomiting, flushing and increased heart rate. These groups tend to consume less alcohol and are at lower risk for alcoholism. In contrast, Native Americans, with a high incidence of alcoholism, generally do not become intoxicated as quickly as other races and therefore may tend to drink more (Thompson & MacDonald 1989).

Religious practices and norms also influence drug taking and drinking practices. The Judeo-Christian traditions accept alcohol use for social purposes while Islam, Buddhism and Sikhism prohibit its consumption. However, Subhra and Chauhan (1999) point to the fact that although certain groups of different ethnic communities place restrictions on the use of alcohol (for religious or cultural reasons), there already exist complex patterns of alcohol use within these communities.

Prevalence and patterns of alcohol and drug misuse

It is estimated that 26 million people worldwide, equivalent to about 0.6% of the global population aged 15–64 years, are problem drug users, and one in every 20 people have tried drugs at least once in the past year (UNODC 2008). Illicit psychoactive substances cause the deaths of 200000 people a year worldwide, and tobacco smoking about 5 million. Around 17.5 million young Europeans (aged 15–34 years) are estimated to have used cannabis in the last year. Some 4 million European adults (aged 15–64 years) are estimated to be using cannabis on a daily basis (EMCDDA 2009). Stimulant drugs such as amphetamines, ecstasy and cocaine are the second most commonly consumed drug type in Europe. Some 12 million adult Europeans have tried cocaine in their lifetime, compared with around 11 million for amphetamines and 9.5 million for ecstasy.

Opioids remain at the heart of Europe's drug phenomenon, with an estimate of between 1.3 and 1.7 million problem opioid users, and account for 50–80% of all treatment demands (EMCDDA 2009). It is estimated that some 3000 new cases of drug-related HIV occur every year in Europe and about 40% of injectors are infected with hepatitis virus C. Drug use varies from region to region, with London and the north of England showing the highest rates, particularly among young people. In general, levels of drug use are higher in deprived areas and council and inner city housing estates.

Alcohol, a favourite drug worldwide, is consumed by approximately 2 billion people and over 76 million people have alcohol use disorders. In most parts of the world the burden related to alcohol consumption in terms of morbidity, mortality and disability is substantial (WHO 2007). The World Health Organization (WHO) estimates that the harmful use of alcohol causes about 2.3 million premature deaths per year worldwide (3.7% of global mortality) and is responsible for 4.4% of the global burden of disease. Although there are regional and national differences in the levels, patterns and contexts of drinking, current trends suggest availability and consumption will continue to rise. The patterns of global alcohol consumption are showing recent increases in consumption in low- and middle-income countries in Southeast Asia and the western Pacific regions. There are worrying concerns that the alcohol industry is rapidly infiltrating the markets of Brazil, India, China and Russia (Editorial 2009). WHO is in the midst of developing a strategy to reduce the harmful use of alcohol, in consultation and collaboration with member states.

The misuse of prescribed psychoactive drugs is also widespread and this has been made more possible by the increasing use of the World Wide Web as a global drug market. Despite efforts by the international law enforcement agencies to close down thousands of illegal Internet pharmacies involved in drug trafficking, there is an increasing number of Internet sites selling medicines containing opioids and stimulants without prescriptions (INCB 2009). The Council for Involuntary Tranquilliser Addiction (CITA), run by Liverpool University, guesstimates that there are as many as 1.5 million nervous types in the UK who have become accidentally addicted to benzodiazepines. According to Ashton (2002), benzodiazepines are now part of the drug scene and are taken illicitly in high doses by 90% of drug misusers worldwide. There is also concern arising from the misuse of 'OTCs', an abbreviation for painkillers bought 'over the counter'. It is estimated that there might be 50 000 OTC addicts in Britain today.

The prescription drugs causing most concern are antidepressants such as Prozac and the newcomers Efexor and Cymbalta. These are classed as selective serotonin and noradrenaline reuptake inhibitors or SSNRIs. These drugs do not simply increase levels of serotonin, the brain chemical that makes us feel more sociable and relaxed, they also boost adrenaline, making us more energetic and sometimes slightly manic.

The alcohol and drug scenes today

In the twentieth century there is no lack of interest in the use of psychoactive substances and plants and new synthetic drugs. In the 1880s few restrictions were places on psychoactive substances such as opium, morphine, cannabis, cocaine and heroin, and these drugs were legal and fairly accessible. Patterns of drug use and misuse frequently change as a result of political and socioeconomic conditions and the same 'old' drugs may reappear in different forms or as so-called 'designer drugs'. These days, the above mentioned psychoactive substances are all under legal control or medical restrictions. In the past, most of the 'old' drugs such as cannabis, tobacco and alcohol were used for religious or medicinal purposes, whereas they are now primarily used as part of recreational and social activities.

The anti-drug stance and the 'war on drugs' have had little effect on the proliferation of psychoactive substances (Rassool 2009). When the United Nations General Assembly special session on drugs was convened in 1998, it committed to 'eliminating or significantly reducing the illicit cultivation of the coca bush, the cannabis plant and the opium poppy by the year 2008' and to 'achieving significant and measurable results in the field of demand reduction'. In 2007, there were still signs of overall stability in the production, trafficking and consumption of cocaine, heroin, cannabis and amphetamines. Whether a 'drug-free world', which the United Nations describes as a realistic goal, is attainable remains to be seen. The year 2008 remains a milestone for international drug control as over 100 years have passed since the first international drug control conference, the 1909 International Opium Commission in Shanghai (UNODC 2009). Today, at an international level, there is a high level of consensus on drug control.

The recent report on world drug trends (UNODC 2008) shows that the recent stabilisation in the world drugs market is under threat. There has been a surge in opium and coca cultivation, and the risk of higher drug use in developing countries threatens to undermine recent progress in drug control. In contrast to the extent of use and mortality statistics of tobacco smoking, only 0.6% of the adult population can be classified as problem drug users (UNODC 2008). In 2007, opium cultivation increased in both Afghanistan and Myanmar. With regard to cocaine, cultivation increased in Bolivia, Peru and especially Colombia, but yields declined, so production remained stable. Although the cannabis market is stable, Afghanistan has become a major producer of cannabis resin, perhaps exceeding Morocco. Indoor cultivation of cannabis is a growing business in developed countries, and more potent strains of cannabis herb are being produced. In 2007, global amphetamine-type stimulant (ATS) production increased slightly but there was a decline in both ecstasy and methamphetamine productions. Khat is a stimulant that is used in Somalia, Ethiopia, Kenya and the Yemeni republics. Although illegal in most European countries and the USA, it is legal in the UK. Whilst khat use in its natural form may not present a significant social and health problem, a potent synthetic form of active ingredients may cause severe social, psychological, physical and economic harms to the individual and to their families and communities.

In Europe, one of the recent concerns regarding the use of psychoactive herbal mixture is illustrated, for example, by the use of 'Spice'. Spice refers to a blend of plant or herbal ingredients, including Indian Warrior and Lion's Tail (EMCDDA 2009). Different blends and flavours are marketed under a variety of names, including: Spice silver, Spice gold, Spice diamond, Spice tropical synergy and Spice Yucatan fire. Some users have reported that, when smoked, Spice products can have similar effects to those produced by cannabis. A number of Spice products can be bought on the Internet and in smartshops and sold as a mix of air-refreshing herbs. Some countries of the European Union have taken legal action to ban or otherwise control Spice products.

Policy initiatives and strategies

Despite the long-standing political prominence of the problem, relatively coherent strategies and substantial investment, the UK remains at the top of the European ladder with the highest level of dependent and recreational drug use (UKDCP 2007). Since the 1990s, the UK government has responded to high-profile alcohol and drug problems with various policies and initiatives. The UK government has adopted a comprehensive demand reduction strategy to tackle alcohol and drug misuse through various policies and guidelines and has scored some significant successes. With the introduction of the National Treatment Agency for Substance Misusers, the purpose is to double the number of people in effective, well-managed treatment and to increase the proportion of people completing or appropriately continuing treatment, year on year. The government's wider national drugs strategy sets out a harm reduction approach to reducing the number of drug-related deaths and blood-borne virus infections.

The 2007 clinical guidelines (Department of Health 2007) focus on drug treatment effectiveness, principles of clinical governance, essential elements of treatment provision, psychosocial components of treatment, health considerations and specific treatment situations and populations. The *Models of Care for Treatment of Adult Drug Misusers* or *MoCDM* (NTA 2002) sets out a national framework, in England, for the commissioning of adult treatment for drug misuse to meet the needs of diverse local populations and to improve the quality and effectiveness of drug treatment. The 2006 update (NTA 2006) is intended to build on the framework and concepts in *MoCDM 2002* rather than replace them. *MoDCM Updated 2006* also incorporates a new strategy to improve the quality and effectiveness of drug treatment. The *Models of Care for Alcohol Misusers* or *MoCAM* (NTA 2007) sets a framework for the development of structured treatment and integrated care pathways for those who misuse alcohol. A recent 10-year drug strategy (2008–2018) (Home Office 2008) aims to restrict the supply of illegal drugs and reduce the demand for them. It focuses on protecting families and strengthening communities. The four strands of work within the strategy are:

1 Protecting communities through tackling drug supply, drug-related crime and anti-social behaviour.
2 Preventing harm to children, young people and families affected by drug misuse.
3 Delivering new approaches to drug treatment and social re-integration.
4 Public information campaigns, communications and community engagement.

The government's wider national drugs strategy is to reduce drug-related deaths due to overdose and blood-borne viruses. Blood-borne virus infections can cause chronic poor health and can lead to serious disease and premature death.

The Alcohol Harm Reduction Strategy for England (Prime Minister's Strategy Unit 2007) is a coherent strategy that sets out the government's aims for reducing alcohol-related harm and costs of alcohol misuse. The strategy recognises the need for coordination of services and commits to working within the 'Models of care' framework on integrated care pathways. It also has a series of measures that aim to tackle alcohol-related disorder in town and city centres, improve treatment and support for people with alcohol problems, clamp down on irresponsible promotions by the industry, and provide better information to consumers about the dangers of alcohol misuse.

Conclusions

Society has learned to coexist with drugs and alcohol. It is stated that drug problems will not be beaten out of society by yet harsher laws, lectured out of society by yet more hours of 'health education', or treated out of society by yet more drug experts (Royal College of Psychiatrists 1989). Addiction is now regarded as a global public health problem. Addiction to alcohol and drugs is associated with health problems, poverty, violence, criminal behaviour and social exclusion. It is envisaged that a comprehensive response to addiction is through the implementation of both prevention and treatment strategies. Demand and harm reduction strategies are of global public health importance. A comprehensive package needs to include efforts to stop or reduce production and trafficking of illicit drugs (supply reduction) combined with the prevention of drug use and treatment and harm reduction.

Summary of key points

- Alcohol and drug misuse remain a global health problem.
- We are all addicted to something, whether it is alcohol or drugs, chocolate, texting on mobile phones, jogging or watching soap operas on TV.
- The nature and extent of the problem will depend upon the individual, the type of psychoactive active substance(s) used and the environment.
- From the earliest times, alcohol and drugs have been used for medicinal, religious, cultural and recreational purposes and as a social lubricant.
- Alcohol has been used for pleasure, nutrition, medicine, ritual, remuneration and funerary purposes.
- Opium is an extract of the exudates derived from seed pods of the opium poppy.
- During the last four decades, cannabis remains the most frequently used illicit drug in the UK.
- Morphine was used for the treatment of opium addiction.
- LSD was primarily used as an adjunct to psychotherapy, in the treatment of alcoholism, drug dependence, sexual problems and psychotic and neurotic disorders.
- Tobacco was believed to be a cure-all, and was used to dress wounds, as well as a painkiller for toothache.
- Drug controls have enabled a stabilisation in the proliferation of psychoactive substances.

References

Aston H. (2002) *Benzodiazepines: how they work and how to withdraw*. School of Neurosciences, Royal Victoria Infirmary, Newcastle upon Tyne: http://www.benzo.org.uk/manual/.

Bloomquist E.R. (1971) *Marijuana: the second trip*, revised edn. Glencoe Press, Beverly Hills, CA.

Department of Health (2007) *Drug Misuse and Dependence: guidelines on clinical management*. HMSO, London.

Editorial (2009) Editorial. Alcohol misuse needs a global response. *Lancet*, 373(9662), 433. doi:10.1016/S0140-6736(09)60146.

EMCDDA (European Monitoring Centre for Drugs and Drug Addiction) (2009) *Drugnet Europe*. Newsletter of the EMCDDA, January–March 2009: Emcdda.europa.eu.

Ghodse A.H. (1995) *Drugs and Addictive Behaviour. A guide to treatment*. Blackwell Science, Oxford.

Gossop M. (1989) *Living with Drugs*. Wilwood Publications, Aldershot.

Home Office (2008) *Drugs: protecting families and communities – 2008–2018 strategy*. Home Office, London: http://drugs.homeoffice.gov.uk/drug-strategy/overview/.

Imperial Tobacco Canada (2007) *Tobacco History 2007*. www.imperialtobaccocanada.com (accessed 24 March 2009).

INCB (2007) Report of the International Narcotics Control Board for 2006, United Nations Publication, New York, 2007 E/INCB/2006/1. http://www.incb.org/pdf/e/ar/2006/annual-report-2006-en.pdf.

Johnson M.R.D. & Carroll M. (1995) *Dealing with Diversity: good practice in drug prevention work with racially and culturally diverse communities*. Centre for Research in Ethnic Relations, University of Warwick.

Kohn M. (1992) *Dope Girls. The birth of the British drug underground*. Lawrence & Wishart, London.

Lewin L. (1964) *Phantastica: narcotic and stimulating drugs – their use and abuse*. Routledge & Kegan Paul, London.

NTA (National Treatment Agency) (2002) *Models of Care for Treatment of Adult Drug Misusers. Parts 1 and 2*. NTA Publications, London.

NTA (National Treatment Agency) (2006) *Models of Care for Treatment of Adult Drug Misusers Updated*. NTA Publications, London.

NTA (National Treatment Agency) (2007) *Models of Care for Alcohol Misusers*. Department of Health, London.

Petersen R.C. (1977) History of cocaine. In R.C. Petersen & R.C. Stillman (eds) *Cocaine*, pp. 17–34. Research Monograph No. 13. National Institute of Drug Abuse, Washington, DC.

Rassool G.H. (2009) *Alcohol and Drug Misuse. A handbook for student and health professionals*. Routledge, London.

Royal College of Psychiatrists (1989) *Drug Scenes. A report on drugs and drug dependence*. Gaskell, London.

Stevens J. (1987) *Storming Heaven: LSD and the American dream*. Atlantic Monthly Press, New York.

Subhra G. & Chauhan V. (1999) *Developing Black Services: an evaluation of the African, Caribbean and Asian services*. Alcohol Concern, London.

Prime Minister's Strategy Unit (2007) *Alcohol Harm Reduction Strategy for England*. Cabinet Office, London: http://www.cabinetoffice.gov.uk/strategy/work_areas/alcohol_misuse.aspx (accessed 20 December 2008).

Thompson P.R. & MacDonald J.L. (1989) Multicultural health education: responding to the challenge. *Health Promotion*, 8(11).

UKDPC (UK Drug Policy Commission) (2007) *An Analysis of UK Drug Policy*. UKDPC, London: www.ukdpc.org.uk.

UNODC (United Nations Drugs Office and Crime) (2007) *World Drug Report 2007*. UNODC, Vienna: http://www.unodc.org/pdf/research/wdr07/WDR_2007_executive_summary.pdf (accessed 24 March 2009).

UNODC (United Nations Drugs Office and Crime) (2008) *World Drug Report 2008*. UNODC, Vienna: http://www.unodc.org/documents/wdr/WDR_2008 (accessed 24 March 2009).

UNODC (United Nations Drugs Office and Crime) (2009) *Annual Report of the United Nations Office on Drugs and Crime*. UNODC, Vienna.

Whitaker B. (1987) *The Global Connection: the crisis of drug addiction*. Jonathan Cape, London.

WHO (World Health Organization) (2007) *WHO Expert Committee on Problems Related to Alcohol Consumption. Second report*. WHO, Geneva.

4 Introduction to Alcohol and Drugs

The language of 'addiction' is confusing and it is essential to have a common language for understanding the complexities of addiction to alcohol and drugs. This chapter presents an explanation of the terminology related to alcohol and drugs, including definitions of the terms such as addiction, drugs, drug misuse, problem drug users and problem drinkers, psychological and physical dependence, and the dependence syndrome.

What is a drug?

A drug can be any sort of food (e.g. chocolate) that affects the way your body functions. The concept of a drug is heavily influenced by the sociocultural context and the purpose of its use. The therapeutic use of a drug means a pharmacological preparation used in the prevention, diagnosis and treatment of an abnormal or pathological condition, whereas the non-therapeutic use of drugs commonly refers to the use of illegal or socially disapproved of substances (Rassool 1998). A drug, in the broadest sense, is a chemical substance that has an effect on bodily systems and behaviour. This includes a wide range of prescribed drugs, illegal drugs and socially accepted substances, and they can be either therapeutic or non-therapeutic, or both. A summary of the terminology related to drugs is presented in Table 4.1.

Addiction for Nurses By G. Hussein Rassool. © 2010 G. Hussein Rassool

Table 4.1 Definitions: addiction and drugs.

Addiction	Addictive behaviour includes the misuse of psychoactive substances and activities leading to excessive behavioural patterns (eating, drinking, drug use, gambling and sexuality)
Drugs	'Any substance or chemical that alters the structure or functioning of a living being' (WHO 1981) The therapeutic use of a drug means a pharmacological preparation used in the prevention, diagnosis and treatment of an abnormal or pathological condition The non-therapeutic use of drugs commonly refers to the use of illegal or socially disapproved substances (Rassool 1998) Drugs, in the context of this book, refer to all psychoactive substances (alcohol, drugs, tobacco) that are licit, illicit and prescribed
Drug misuse	'Drug misuse may be seen as the use of drugs in a socially unacceptable way that is harmful or hazardous to the individual or others' (Royal College of Psychiatrists and Royal College of Physicians Working Party 2000)
Unsanctioned use	A drug that is not approved by society
Hazardous use	A drug leading to harm or dysfunction
Dysfunctional use	A drug leading to impaired psychological or social functioning
Harmful use	A drug that is known to have caused tissue damage or psychiatric disorders
Drug dependence	The behavioural responses that always include a compulsion to take the drug in order to experience its physical or psychological effects, and sometimes to avoid the discomfort of its absence. Dependence is often described as either physical or psychological

Problem drug users and problem drinkers

The terms problem drug user and problem drinker have been used to refer to those who are dependent on psychoactive substances. Table 4.2 provides an explanation of the terms. The definition of problem drug user focuses on the needs and problems of the individual in acknowledging that the problem drug user has social, psychological, physical and legal needs. The definition could be expanded to incorporate the spiritual needs of the problem drug user or problem drinker (Rassool 2001; Hammond & Rassool 2006). In relation to problem drinkers, the same definition for problem drug use is applicable. However, a broader category of those at risk of harmful consequences includes: hazardous drinkers, harmful drinkers, moderately dependent drinkers and severely dependent drinkers.

Hazardous drinkers are drinking at levels over the sensible drinking limits, either in terms of regular excessive consumption or less frequent sessions of heavy

Table 4.2 Definitions: problem drug users and problem drinkers.

Problem drug users	'… any person who experiences social, psychological, physical or legal problems related to intoxication and\or regular excessive consumption and\or dependence as a consequence of his own use of drugs or other chemical substances … and may involve or lead to sharing of injecting equipment' (ACMD 1982, 1988)
Problem drinkers	'… any person who experiences social, psychological, physical or legal problems related to intoxication and/or regular excessive consumption and/or dependence as a consequence of his own use of alcohol. Similar to those described as severely dependent drinkers'
Hazardous	'A pattern of substance use that increases the risk of harmful consequences for the user … hazardous use refers to patterns of use that are of public health significance despite the absence of any current disorder in the individual user' (WHO 1994)
Harmful	'A pattern of use which is already causing damage to health. The damage may be physical or mental' (WHO 1992)
Moderately dependent	'Moderately dependent drinkers may recognise that they have a problem with drinking and they may not have reached the stage of "relief drinking"– which is drinking to relieve or avoid physical discomfort from withdrawal symptoms' (NTA 2006)
Severely dependent	Individuals in this category may have serious and long-standing problems, 'chronic alcoholism', and may have been heavy users over prolonged periods. This habit of significant alcohol consumption may be due in part to preventing withdrawal symptoms

drinking. In the UK, the Department of Health advises that men should not drink more than 3–4 units of alcohol per day, and women should drink no more than 2–3 units of alcohol per day. Harmful drinkers are usually drinking at levels above those recommended for sensible drinking, typically at higher levels than most hazardous drinkers and show clear evidence of some alcohol-related harm. Moderately dependent drinkers or 'chronic alcoholics' may recognise that they have a problem with drinking. Individuals who are severely dependent drinkers may have been heavy users over prolonged periods and have serious and long-standing problems – 'chronic alcoholism'. This group of drinkers may have complex needs such as coexisting psychiatric problems, learning disabilities, poly-drug use or complicated assisted alcohol withdrawal.

Psychological and physical dependence

Table 4.3 provides an explanation of tolerance, psychological dependence, physical dependence and withdrawal. Individuals can develop tolerance to a variety of psychoactive substances but the drug must be taken on a regular basis and in adequate quantities for tolerance to occur. For example, amphetamines can

Table 4.3 Psychological and physical dependence.

Tolerance	Tolerance refers to the way the body usually adapts to the repeated presence of a drug. Higher quantities or doses of the psychoactive substance are required to reproduce the desired or similar cognitive, affective or behavioural effects. Individuals can develop tolerance to a variety of psychoactive substances. Tolerance may develop rapidly in the case of LSD (lysergic acid diethylamide) or slowly in the case of alcohol or opiates
Psychological dependence	Psychological dependence can be described as a compulsion or a craving to continue to take the substance because of the need for stimulation, or because it relieves anxiety or depression. Psychological dependence is recognised as the most widespread and most important type of dependence
Physical dependence	Physical dependence is characterised by the need to take a psychoactive substance to avoid physical disturbances or withdrawal symptoms following cessation of use. The withdrawal symptoms depend on the type or category of drug(s)
Withdrawal	Withdrawal refers to the wide range of symptoms that occur after stopping or dramatically reducing alcohol or opiate drugs after heavy and prolonged use (several weeks or more). If a physically dependent user does not take a repeat dose they suffer physical withdrawal symptoms

produce considerable tolerance and strong psychological dependence with little or no physical dependence, and cocaine can produce psychological dependence without tolerance or physical dependence.

Psychological dependence is accepted as the most widespread and the most important. However, it is not only attributed to the use of psychoactive drugs but also to food, sex, gambling, relationships or physical activities. In physical dependence, there is a need to take alcohol or the drug to avoid withdrawal symptoms following cessation of use. The severity of the withdrawal symptoms depends on the type or category of the psychoactive substances. For example, withdrawal from alcohol can cause hallucinations or epileptic fits and may be life threatening, whereas the physiological withdrawal symptoms from nicotine abstinence may be relatively slight. In other dependence-inducing psychoactive substances such as opiates and depressants the withdrawal experience can range from mild to severe. It is possible to have dependence without withdrawal and withdrawal without dependence (Royal College of Psychiatrists 1987). Many of the supposed signs of physical dependence are sometimes psychosomatic reactions triggered

Table 4.4   The dependence syndrome.

■ Increased tolerance to the drug
■ Repeated withdrawal symptoms
■ Compulsion to use the drug (psychological state known as craving)
■ Salience of drug-seeking behaviour (obtaining and using the drug become more important in the person's life)
■ Relief or avoidance of withdrawal symptoms (regular use of the drug to relieve withdrawal symptoms)
■ Narrowing of the repertoire of drug taking (pattern of drinking may become an everyday activity)
■ Rapid reinstatement after abstinence

Source: Edwards G. & Gross, M. (1976) Alcohol dependence: provisional description of a clinical syndrome. *British Journal of Addiction*, 81, 171–173.

not by the chemical properties of the psychoactive drug but by the user's fears, beliefs and fantasies about what withdrawal entails (Plant 1987).

The dependence syndrome

The Tenth Revision of the International Classification of Diseases and Health Problems (ICD-10) defines the dependence syndrome as being a cluster of physiological, behavioural and cognitive phenomena in which the use of a substance or a class of substances takes on a much higher priority for a given individual than other behaviours that once had greater value. The significant characteristic includes the desire (often strong, sometimes overpowering) to take the psychoactive drug. Although the original framework of the dependence syndrome referred specifically to alcohol dependence, this has been expanded to include other psychoactive substances. According to Edwards and Gross (1976), there are seven components of the syndrome (Table 4.4).

How people take drugs (routes of drug administration)

There are several routes of administration of psychoactive substances: orally, smoking, inhalation and by injection (Table 4.5). The speed of onset of the physical and psychological effects of the drug depends upon its route of administration. The most common route of administration is orally, in either liquid or tablet form. When a drug is required to act more rapidly. the preferred route of administration is by injection. Heroin, for example, is often administered intravenously, for example directly into a vein. Certain drugs are smoked, for example cannabis, crack cocaine and heroin. Some psychoactive drugs, for example cocaine and amphetamines, are also taken by the intranasal route. The complications of injecting are presented in Table 4.6.

Table 4.5 Routes of drug administration.

Oral (swallowing)	■ Most popular method of drug administration ■ The slowest route because of the slow absorption of the drug into the blood stream ■ No stigma attached, compared to smoking and injecting
Smoking	■ Effective route where the drug is inhaled ■ For example, tobacco or heroin smoking ('chasing the dragon')
Inhalation (sniffing)	■ Absorption of the drug is through the mucous membrane of the nose and mouth ■ The type of drugs that are inhaled includes cocaine, tobacco snuff and volatile substances and solvents
Injecting	■ Methods of drug injecting include intramuscularly or subcutaneously and/or intravenously ■ Injection of drugs is less widespread than other routes of drug administration but also the most hazardous ■ The major danger of injecting is the risk of overdose because of the concentrated effect of this method ■ There is also the risk of infection from non-sterile injection methods including hepatitis B and HIV (human immunodeficiency virus) infections, abscesses, gangrene and thromboses ■ The onset of the effects of the drug is rapid when it is administered intravenously and is a major reason why drugs are often self-administered by injection

Table 4.6 Complications of injecting.

Equipment	Drug	Site of injection	Effects
General environment	Type of drug	Trauma and infection:	Overdose
Cooker/water/filter	Drug interactions	Skin abscess	Poisoning
Water	Allergy	Fat necrosis	Infection
Filter	Contaminants	'Simple' miss	Thrombosis
Syringe	Infectious agents	Connective tissue	Embolism
Needles		Arterial injection	
		Nerves	
		Lungs, breasts, penis, neck	

Source: adapted from Pates R., McBride A. & Arnold K. (2005) *Injecting Illicit Drugs*, p. xiii. Blackwell, Oxford.

Summary of key points

■ Drug use includes a wide range of prescribed drugs, illegal substances and socially accepted substances.
■ The terms problem drug user and problem drinker have been used to refer to those who are dependent on psychoactive substances.
■ Individuals can develop tolerance to a variety of psychoactive substances.
■ Dependence has two components: physical and psychological dependence.
■ Drugs can produce considerable tolerance and strong psychological dependence with little or no physical dependence.
■ The withdrawal symptoms depend on the type or category of drugs used.
■ The routes of administration are oral, smoking, inhalation and injection.
■ Injecting drugs is less widespread than other routes of drug administration but also the most hazardous.

References

ACMD (Advisory Council on the Misuse of Drugs) (1982) *Treatment and Rehabilitation*. HMSO, London.

ACMD (Advisory Council on the Misuse of Drugs) (1988) *Aids and Drug Misuse: Part 1*. HMSO, London.

Edwards G. & Gross, M. (1976) Alcohol dependence: provisional description of a clinical syndrome. *British Journal of Addiction*, 81, 171–173.

Hammond A. & Rassool G.H. (2006) Spiritual and cultural needs: integration in dual diagnosis care. In G.H. Rassool (ed.) *Dual Diagnosis Nursing*, pp. 209–221. Blackwell Publishing, Oxford.

NTA (National Treatment Agency) (2006) *Models of Care for Alcohol Misusers (MoCAM)*. NTA, London.

Pates R., McBride A. & Arnold K. (2005) *Injecting Illicit Drugs*. Blackwell, Oxford.

Plant M. (1987) *Drugs in Perspective*. Hodder & Stoughton, London.

Rassool G.H. (1998) *Substance Use and Misuse: nature, context and clinical interventions*. Blackwell Science, Oxford.

Rassool G.H. (2001) Substance use and dual diagnosis: concepts, theories and models. In G.H. Rassool (ed.) *Dual Diagnosis: substance misuse and psychiatric disorders*, pp. 12–32. Blackwell Science, Oxford.

Royal College of Psychiatrist (1987) *Drug Scenes. A report on drugs and drug dependence*. Royal College of Psychiatrists/Gaskell, London.

Royal College of Psychiatrists and Royal College of Physicians Working Party (2000) *Drugs: Dilemmas and Choices*. Gaskell, London.

WHO (World Health Organization) (1981) Nomenclature and classification of drug- and alcohol-related problems: a WHO memorandum. *Bulletin of the World Health Organization*, 59, 225–242.

WHO (World Health Organization) (1992) *International Classification of Diseases: the ICD-10 Classification of Mental and Behavioural Disorders (ICD-10)*. WHO, Geneva.

WHO (World Health Organization) (1994) *Lexicon of Alcohol and Drug Terms*. WHO, Geneva.

5 Nature and Pattern of Addiction

This chapter examines the drug experience, why people take drugs, and the pattern of use and misuse.

The drug experience

It is important to note that, whatever the level of use, drugs affect different people in different ways. The effects that a psychoactive substance or 'drug experience' will have on a given individual will depend on several other factors beside the pharmacological properties of the drug, such as the set and the setting. The set is the personality or the psychological state an individual brings to the experience, like thoughts, mood or expectations. The setting refers to the context of the physical or social environment. Table 5.1 presents an outline of the drug experience.

The pharmacological factors include the chemical properties or type of drug used. Different drugs have different mode of action on the body due to their pharmacological properties; also important is the purity and strength of the drug, the route of administration and whether it is used in combination with other drugs. In addition, the effects or actions of a psychoactive drug are influenced by

Addiction for Nurses By G. Hussein Rassool. © 2010 G. Hussein Rassool

Table 5.1 The drug experience.

Pharmacological factors	▦ Chemical properties of the drug ▦ Different drugs have different modes of action on the body ▦ Drug dosage ▦ Route of administration
Individual (set)	▦ Physical factors: body weight, sex, race, current health conditions, diseases, medication intake and genetic inheritance ▦ Level of experience with the particular drug ▦ Tolerance influenced by level of experience and physical factors (body weight) ▦ Current emotional and mental state (depression, anger, stress. recent trauma) ▦ Type and level of drug education received ▦ Expectations (or lack of), as well as intentions, regarding the effects and experiences of the drug used ▦ Personality factors
Context (setting)	▦ Environment where the drug taking occurs ▦ Time, such as day or night ▦ Communication and interaction ▦ Culture and rituals ▦ Reason for drug experience

the personal characteristics of the drug user. These characteristics include factors such as the person's biological make-up, personality, gender, age and drug tolerance (Rassool 1998) and the user's previous experience of the drug. The psychological state of the individual is also relevant, for example those with low mood or who are anxious or depressed are more liable to have disturbing experiences when using psychoactive substances. Health problems such as cardiovascular disease, hypertension, asthma, epilepsy, diabetes mellitus or liver disease can exacerbate the use of psychoactive substances and make them more unsafe. The last set of factors to be considered is the setting or context in which a drug is used. This includes the physical environment where the drug is used, the cultural influences of the community where the drug is consumed, the laws relating to drug use and the context in which a drug is used. It is stated that 'it is necessary to see the drug–brain interaction not as a simple chemical event but as a matter of considerable complexity involving the drug, the particular person, and the messages and teachings which come from the environment and which powerfully influence the nature and meaning of the drug experience' (Royal College of Psychiatrists 1987).

All the three interrelated factors – pharmacological properties, individual differences (set) and context of use (setting) – influence the individual experiences of drug taking.

Why do people use drugs?

Psychoactive substances cause a series of temporary changes in the nervous system that produce a feeling of being 'high'. There are several factors that might put someone at risk for drug use. These risk factors can be found at the individual, family, peer group and broader community levels. Research on the pathways from no use to alcohol and drug misuse suggests the immediate decision to use drugs is driven, basically, by one of two types of reasons. Individuals who use drugs, including alcohol, do so because they enjoy it and they like the 'high' that is produced by the substances. In fact, the subjective initial experiences of taking psychoactive substances are often pleasurable. There is a tendency to seek fun and novelty in drug taking. Users may be attracted to illicit drugs for similar reasons as they are to alcohol. Furthermore, the use of drugs for pleasure is readily identifiable throughout history and across most cultures (Siegel 2005).

Another group of individuals use drugs for quite different purposes: they self-medicate in order to feel better and to cope with difficult life situations. This group of individuals may also be suffering from emotional and psychosocial problems. Environmental risk factors are a major influence on an individual's surroundings that increase the likelihood of that person using psychoactive substances. Drug and alcohol misuse tend to thrive in areas of multiple deprivation, with high unemployment and low-quality housing and where the surrounding infrastructure of local services is fractured and poorly resourced. However, substance misuse is certainly not restricted to areas of urban deprivation. Curiosity, the subset of youth culture and music, social acceptability, peer pressure and the media can also promote drug use. A list of the reasons why people use drugs is presented in Table 5.2.

Table 5.2 Reasons why people use drugs.

■ To enjoy the experience	■ To counter the unpleasant effects of prescribed medications
■ To get the same experience as from alcohol	■ To continue the habit
■ To enjoy the short-term effects	■ It is part of one's home/social life
■ To feel confident	■ To relieve boredom
■ To 'break the rules'	■ To alleviate pain
■ To be part of the subculture	■ To satisfy cravings
■ Curiosity about the effects	■ To avoid withdrawal symptoms
■ The drugs are easily accessible and available	■ To counter the withdrawal effects of other drugs (e.g. use of benzodiazepines after stimulants)
■ Their friends use them	■ To lose weight
■ To avoid unpleasant feelings	■ To escape from stress
■ To enhance work performances	

The reason why people start using drugs may not be the same as the reason why they continue to use them. Continued use of psychoactive substances is influenced more by physical and psychological addiction. The reasons why people continue to use drugs may be related to a combination of factors such as dependence, chaotic use, fear of withdrawal symptoms, social exclusions, mental health problems and other psychosocial and environmental conditions.

Patterns of substance use and misuse

The pattern of substance misuse reflects a broad spectrum, ranging from no use to dependence. These patterns, for some individuals, may vary over a period of time and are often described as no use, and experimental, recreational and problematic use. Individuals may move back and forth within this continuum, but generally they advance from no use, to use, misuse and finally to dependence (Table 5.3).

In the no use stage there is no use of alcohol or other drugs. Individuals have their own reasons not to be involved in alcohol and drug use. Experimental users can be described as those who have used drugs, legal or illicit, on a few occasions. By definition, anyone's initial use of a drug, alcohol or tobacco smoking is experimental (Rassool 1998). The choice of drug used depends on factors such as availability, social marketing, reputation of the drug, subculture, fashion and peer group influence. The motivating factors include curiosity, a desire to share a social experience, anticipation of effects, availability and value for money (cost of drug). This stage usually forms part of the desire among adolescents to experiment and try new, risky experiences and can be seen as a normal developmental pattern. What is unclear is the likelihood of future engagement with, or disengagement from, further alcohol and drug use.

The term 'recreational' refers to a form of substance use in which pleasure and relaxation are the prime motivations. Generally, recreational users refrain from using hard drugs as a result of their personal calculations of risk and pleasure. Recreational users, however, are also in the highest category of risk for infections. Some recreational drugs act as sexual stimulants, lowering inhibition and increasing sexual drive, which often leads to risky sexual behaviour and increased likelihood of HIV (human immunodeficiency virus) infection. A dependent user has progressed to problematic use of a psychoactive drug. There is a high degree of tolerance and there is the presence of psychological and\or physical dependence. Personal, social, psychological and legal problems may be present in this group.

Chaotic use

Chaotic use is referred to when an individual is regarded as taking a drug or drugs in a spontaneous way that tends not to follow any typical drug-using pattern. It

Table 5.3 Patterns of alcohol and drug use.

No use	▣ In this stage there is no use of alcohol or other drugs ▣ People have their own reasons not to be involved, including religious beliefs, their age, the criminal justice system etc.
Experimental use	▣ Drugs, legal or illicit, are used on a few occasions ▣ Anyone's initial use of a drug, alcohol or tobacco smoking is experimental (Rassool 1998) ▣ Users have a low tolerance to the drug ▣ There is no 'pattern' in the use of psychoactive substances but the choice of the drug misused is indiscriminate ▣ The use of psychoactive substances is usually unplanned ▣ This category has the highest risk for infections (if injecting), medical complications or overdose due to the indiscriminate use of adulterated psychoactive substances
Recreational use	▣ The term 'recreational' refers to a form of substance use in which pleasure and relaxation are the prime motivations. The most common drugs used are alcohol, caffeine, nicotine, cannabis, LSD and ecstasy ▣ Drug or alcohol use is one aspect of the user's life and tends to complement social and recreational activities ▣ There are usually no adverse medical or social consequences as a result of the recreational use, as in the case of controlled drinking ▣ Recreational users, however, are also in the highest category of risk for infections
Dependent use	▣ A dependent user has progressed to regular and problematic use of a psychoactive drug or has become a poly-drug user (multiple drug use) ▣ Tolerance is very high and there is the presence of psychological and\or physical dependence thus distinguishing it from experimental and recreational use ▣ The pattern of use is more frequent and regular but less controlled, and is continued despite negative consequences ▣ Injecting drugs is common, and the frequent use creates problems of intoxication, infections if sharing needles and syringes, and other medical complications ▣ Personal, social, psychological and legal problems may be present in this group

is generally associated with problematic bouts of heavy use that may cause the user harm (Drugscope 2007). Basically, the individual in this state focuses more on getting hold of the drugs and taking them and neglects their health behaviour. The individual's life is circumscribed by their drug use in completely unordered and unpredictable ways and is combined with other significant health issues such as HIV, liver damage and mental health problems (Rassool 2009). Chaotic users often indulge in the excessive use of multiple drugs or poly-drug use over a prolonged period of time.

Binge drinking

In recent years, the term 'binge drinking' has gained currency as referring to a high intake of alcohol in a single drinking occasion. A government postnote (POST 2005) refers to binge drinking as the consumption of excessive amounts of alcohol within a limited time period. Such behaviour leads to a rapid increase in blood alcohol concentration (BAC) and consequently to drunkenness. Binge drinking has also been defined as the consumption of more than a certain number of drinks over a short period of time, a single drinking session or during a single day (men consuming at least 8, and women at least 6 standard units of alcohol) (Institute of Alcohol Studies 2004).

The features of binge drinking (MCM Research 2004) are:

■ Drinking with the intention of getting drunk, often mixing drinks.
■ Drinking to the point at where the user loses control.
■ Drinking as much as possible in a short space of time.
■ Occasional heavy drinking.

A much simpler definition of binge drinking is drinking too much alcohol over a short period of time, and is usually the type of drinking that leads to drunkenness (Alcohol Concern 2007).

It is well known that binge drinkers are at increased risk of accidents, alcohol poisoning, unsafe sex and having poor social behaviour. Binge drinking and severe intoxication can cause muscular incoordination, blurred vision, stupor, hypothermia, convulsions, depressed reflexes, respiratory depression, hypotension and coma. Death can occur from respiratory or circulatory failure or if binge drinkers inhale their own vomit (Institute of Alcohol Studies 2004). These patterns of behaviour are also relevant to the episodic use of a psychoactive drug, other than alcohol, in large quantities over a period of time, followed by limited use or abstinence.

Harm

Harm caused by substance misuse includes physical harm, social harm, psychological harm and economic harm. Harmful substances are currently regulated according to classification systems (Misuse of Drugs Act) that purport to relate to the harms and risks of each drug. Some drugs are more harmful than others. A new 'matrix of harm' for drugs of abuse has been proposed by Nutt *et al.* (2007). The study proposes that drugs should be classified by the amount of harm that

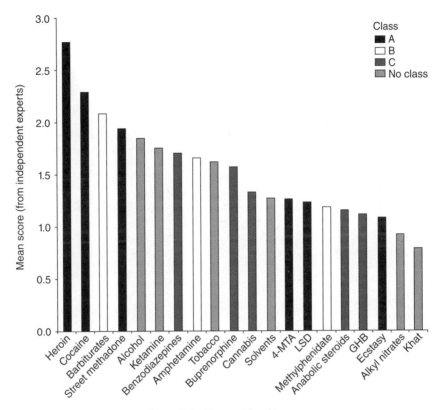

Figure 5.1 The matrix of harm.

they do, rather than the sharp A, B and C divisions used in the UK Misuse of Drugs Act. Nutt *et al.* (2007) identified three main factors that together determine the harm associated with any drug of potential abuse:

1 The physical harm to the individual user caused by the drug.
2 The tendency of the drug to induce dependence.
3 The effect of drug use on families, communities and society.

The new ranking places alcohol and tobacco in the upper half of the league table. These socially accepted drugs were judged more harmful than cannabis, and substantially more dangerous than the class A drugs LSD (lysergic acid diethylamide), 4-MTA (4-methylthioamphetamine) and ecstasy (Figure 5.1). Heroin and cocaine were ranked most dangerous, followed by barbiturates and street methadone. Alcohol was the fifth most harmful drug and tobacco the ninth. Cannabis came in 11th, and near the bottom of the list was ecstasy.

Summary of key points

■ All three interrelated factors – pharmacological properties, individual differences and context of use – influence the individual experiences of drug taking.
■ The patterns of drug or alcohol use/misuse for some individuals vary over a period of time.
■ Continued substance use among alcohol and drug users is driven more by physiological and psychological dependence than by rational decisions.
■ Experimental use of illicit psychoactive substance is usually a short-lived experience and the majority of people confine their consumption to drugs that are socially acceptable.
■ A dependent user has progressed to regular and problematic use of one or more psychoactive drugs.
■ Binge drinking is drinking with the intention of getting drunk.
■ Chaotic use is referred to when an individual is regarded as taking a drug or drugs in a spontaneous way that tends not to follow any typical drug-using pattern.
■ Harm caused by substance misuse includes physical harm, social harm, psychological harm and economic harm.

References

Alcohol Concern (2007) *Binge Drinking Factsheet Summary*. Alcohol Concern, London.

Drugscope (2007) *Media Guide Glossary*. Drugscope, London: http://www.drugscope.org.uk/resources/mediaguide/glossary.

Institute of Alcohol Studies (2004) *Binge Drinking: nature, prevalence and causes*. Institute of Alcohol Studies, St Ives, UK.

MCM Research (2004) *WTAG Binge-drinking Research*. MCM Research Ltd, Oxford.

Nutt D., King L.A., Saulsbury W. & Blakemore C. (2007) Development of a rational scale to assess the harm of drugs of potential misuse. *Lancet*, 369(9566), 1047–1053.

POST (Parliamentary Office of Science and Technology) (2005) *Binge Drinking and Public Health*. Postnote No. 224. POST, London: http://www.parliament.uk/documents/upload/POSTpn244.pdf.

Rassool G.H. (1998) *Substance Use and Misuse: nature, context and clinical interventions*. Blackwell Science, Oxford.

Rassool G.H. (2009) *Alcohol and Drug Misuse. A handbook for students and healthcare professionals*. Routledge, London.

Royal College of Psychiatrists (1987) *Drug Scenes. A report on drugs and drug dependence*. Royal College of Psychiatrists/Gaskell, London.

Siegel R. (2005) *Intoxication. The universal drive for mind-altering substances*. Park Street Press, Vermont.

6 Causes and Maintenance of Addiction

This chapter examines the theories and models of addiction in an attempt to explain the reasons for the initiation into substance misuse or why individuals begin to use drugs and the process of addiction. Many models and theories have been proposed to explain the use or misuse of alcohol and drugs and about the causes of substance use. The theories or models include genetic theory, neuroscientific theories, psychoanalytical theory, behavioural theories, social learning theory, personality theory, sociocultural theories and bio-psychosocial theory. However, the reasons why people start using drugs may not be the same as those that determine why they continue to use drugs. It will become apparent that no single theory is sufficient to explain substance use and misuse per se, and that that a range of 'risk factors' has to be considered. These models or theories should not be considered to be definitive accounts nor is any one theory mutually exclusive of any other.

Addiction for Nurses By G. Hussein Rassool. © 2010 G. Hussein Rassool

Moral theory

For some people, addictive behaviours such as drug taking, heavy drinking or gambling are are seen as a sign of moral weakness, bad character or having a weak will. In the moral theory or model, the individual has deviated from acceptable religious and sociocultural norms. According to this theory, individuals are viewed as responsible for the initiation and development of addictive-related problems. The advocate of this theory does not accept that there is any biological basis for addiction and that individuals are responsible for their behavioural choices and their own recovery, which may consist of mainly spiritual interventions. Much of the stigma faced by substance misusers is based on the underlying moral notion that labels anyone with an alcohol or drug habit as a 'bad person', where the 'victim-blaming' approach is evident. The focus of intervention in the control of behaviour is through social disapproval, spiritual guidance, moral persuasion or imprisonment.

Disease theory

The disease theory of addiction maintains that addiction is a disease that is firmly attributed to the genetic/biological make-up of the individual or behavioural processes, or of some combination of the two. This medical/disease approach also implies the adoption of a sick role by substance misusers and individuals are expected to be treated as having a 'disease'. The proponents of this model hold that alcohol or drug addiction is a unique, irreversible and progressive disease that cannot be cured; due to the inability of the individual to control consumption, abstinence is the only option. This theory also implies that recovery can only be sustained through the goal of total abstinence within self-help group movements (underpinning the disease concept of addiction) such as AA, NA and GA (Alcoholics Anonymous, Narcotic Anonymous, Gamblers Anonymous, respectively). However, this model has been subjected to much criticism based on the assumption that addiction is not a disease but rather a behaviour that can be controlled (Heyman 2009).

Neuropharmacological theories

The neuropharmacological theories of addiction require an understanding of the pharmacological effects of drugs on the brain. Psychoactive substances have different actions on the brain based on the reward systems. Basically, the pathways are the mesolimbic–frontocortical dopamine system and the endogeneous opioid system. The first pathway, the mesolimbic–frontocortical dopamine system, is central to processing neural information about significant stimuli and pleasure. Since the mesolimbic pathway is shown to be associated with feelings of reward and desire, this pathway is heavily implicated in neuropharmacological theories of addiction (Diaz 1996). Addiction may be due to due to increased dopamine transmission in the limbic system, each by different mechanisms.

The second pathway, the endogeneous opioid system, involves endogenous opioids (e.g. endorphins, enkephalins and endomorphins) that are involved in the rewarding effects of other psychoactive substances. For example, the light consumption of alcohol stimulates the release of opioid peptides in brain regions that are associated with reward and reinforcement and that mediate, at least in part, the reinforcing effects of ethanol (Gianoulakis 2001). However, heavy alcohol consumption induces a lack of opioids, which may be perceived as opioid withdrawal and may promote alcohol consumption through the mechanisms of negative reinforcement. The integrated function of both systems underlies pleasure and reward. For a more comprehensive explanation of the neuropharmacological theories of addiction, see Nutt (1997), Nutt and Lingford-Hughes (2008) and Vengeliene et al. (2008).

Genetic theory

The genetic model puts forward a genetic predisposition to alcohol or drug addiction. Studies on families, adoption and twins have suggested that alcohol or drug addiction is the result of genetic or induced biological abnormality of a physiological or structural nature. Family studies of problem drinkers suggest that such disorders cluster in families, especially among siblings (Bierut et al. 1998; Merikangas et al. 1998). Problem drinkers have a 50% chance of having at least one member of their family becoming dependent on alcohol and there is a 90% chance of two or more family members being so dependent (Miller 1991). However, in adoption studies, children whose adopted parents were dependent on alcohol were more likely themselves to develop a problem with alcohol, even though their biological parents were not dependent on alcohol (Miller 1991; Heath 1995).

In a study of pairs of twins, by Tsuang et al. (1996), the findings suggested that the likelihood of developing a dependence to opiates or stimulants was influenced more by genetic factors than by shared environmental factors. Some people may experience a less intense reaction to alcoholic beverages and such vulnerable individuals may drink more before feeling intoxicated. Adityanjee and Murray's (1991) review of twin studies of alcoholism and normal drinking looked at a number of studies in a similar culture and racial group and indicated that alcoholism tends to run in families but acknowledged that no one is clear about what it is that may or may not be transmitted through genetic inheritance. However, when evaluating the pattern of inheritance, all studies showed that it is sons and not daughters that are more at risk of developing alcohol disorders.

One aspect of inheritance that is understood is seen in Eskimos, American Indians and Asians, who are genetically predisposed to have a deficiency in the production of acetaldehyde (an enzyme important for alcohol degradation). These groups are hypersensitive to the effects of alcohol and once higher levels of alcohol are reached in their bodily systems they developed a flushing known as 'Asian flushing'. The lack of these enzymes (alcohol dehydrogenase and aldehyde dehydrogenase) makes it more difficult to metabolise alcohol, causing it to accumulate faster in a person's system, and does not allow the alcohol to break down as quickly.

The degree to which genetic factors play a role in addictive behaviour is still unclear and remains to be further investigated.

Psychological theories

There are a number of psychological theories that attempt to explain the causation of addiction and view heavy alcohol and drug use as problem behaviours. A brief overview of selected theories is presented here.

Psychoanalytical theory

Psychoanalytical theory is derived from the work of Freud, based on the components of the self and their functioning during the stages of psychosexual development. Freud made little reference to alcohol disorders in his published works but did suggest that the consumption of alcohol provided relief from the conflict generated by oral fixation or repressed homosexuality. The use of alcohol or drugs (smoking) is related to 'fixation' at the oral stage of development. Early psychoanalytical explanations developed from the belief that addiction stems from unconscious death wishes as a form of 'slow suicide', the notions of conflict between a repressed idea and the defence against it and a deficient ego (Leeds & Morgenstern 1996).

The aetiology of addiction is assumed to develop from conflicts between the id, ego and super ego, fixation at a stage of oral development and the avoidance of pain and anxiety. In order to avoid pain or anxiety, alcohol intoxication is assumed to provide this relief. Individuals with addictive problems have certain psychodynamic characteristics that include problems in affect management, narcissism, object relations, judgement and self-care (Treece & Khantzian 1986). These problems may predispose individuals to drug dependence because they are the basis of anxieties or distresses that are relieved by taking psychoactive substance.

Behavioural theories

In behavioural theories, the use of psychoactive substances is viewed as an acquired behaviour, a response that is learned through the process of classical conditioning (Pavlovian conditioning), operant conditioning (Skinner) and social learning. In classical conditioning, dependence is in part acquired through the process of associative learning. That is, the desire to use drugs may be the result of specific factors associated with the use of a particular substance. Addictive behaviour is maintained by the reinforcers of such behaviour (West 2006).

Reinforcements strengthen behaviour and may be positive (rewarding behaviour) or negative (avoidance of an unpleasant experience). The role of positive reinforcement in the use of psychoactive substances can be explained by the fact that drugs can cause pleasurable sensations. The more pleasure or in some cases fear of withdrawal reinforce the continued use of the substance.

Cue exposure theory, an element of classical conditioning theory, is based on the notion that cues are important in the development and maintenance of addictive behaviour (Drummond *et al.* 1995). Cues occur before the use of psychoactive substances and may include the sight of a needle or syringe, the smell of alcohol, the sight of publicity for alcohol or tobacco, the environment, a depressed mood and beliefs about drug effects (Drummond *et al.* 1995). The maintenance of drug-taking behaviour is the result of past associations with drug-taking environments or situations.

Personality theory

Within the framework of psychological theories, personality theory stresses the importance of personal traits and characteristics in the formation and maintenance of dependence. Traits such as hyperactivity, sensation seeking, antisocial behaviour and impulsivity have been found to be associated with substance misuse (Sher *et al.* 1991). The habit of using psychoactive substances is developed because the drug fulfils a certain purpose that is related to the individual's personality (Eysenck 1997). Studies with adolescents showed that those who are disruptive and have less conformist attitudes were more likely to drink, smoke and use illicit psychoactive substances (Institute of Medicine 1996).

According to Ghodse (1995: 20) while 'there is an epidemiological association between drug misuse and personality disorder, no deductions can be made about causality as most studies have compared drug-dependent with non-dependent individuals'. He asserted that there might be personality traits that change the likelihood of an individual becoming dependent on drugs.

Social learning theory

Social learning theory (or cognitive social learning) provides an explanation of how behaviour (adaptive or maladaptive) is formed and maintained through the process of role modelling and the need to conform (Bandura 1977; Barnes 1990). For example, an individual's consumption of alcohol will vary to match that of a drinking partner and this demonstrates that modelling affects drinking behaviour (Collins & Marlatt 1981). In effect, patterns of behaviour and attitudes can also be acquired through the observation of social models without any reinforcement of overt behaviour.

However, in order to understand the effects of alcohol or drugs, cognitive processes must be considered in relation to other factors. There is also an interrelationship between personal (expectations, beliefs, cognitions) and environmental (context, social setting) factors. That is, an individual's prior experiences with alcohol or drugs and the social setting in which drinking or drug taking occurs must be considered. Orford (1985) proposed a theory of 'excessive appetites' within the context of the social learning paradigm. He developed a theory of addiction and maintained that the degree of an individual's involvement with 'appetitive activities' includes biological, personality, social and ecological determinants.

Sociocultural theories

Sociocultural theories include a number of sub-theories such as systems theory, anomie theory, family interaction theory, anthropological theory, economic theory, gateway theory and availability theory. From a sociological perspective, addiction is described as 'an individual behaviour that has a social effect, it affects other people; it is also an individual behaviour that is controlled at the societal level' (Adrian 2003: 3). Addiction is seen as a socially constructed phenomena and addiction is an adaptation to the divergence between society's culturally defined goals and the socially prescribed means for achieving those goals (Merton 1971). Failure to achieve these goals might relinquish both the goals and the legitimate means for achieving them and lead to escape through drug addiction.

The idea of alcoholism as a 'family disease' or 'family disorder' has been proposed by Steinglass (1987). In the family interaction theory, the most significant aetiological factor is probably parental deficits (e.g. parental absence, family tension, rejection, emotional distancing or parental alienation) that occur as a product of parental alcoholism. There is also some evidence to suggest that alcohol may serve as an adaptive function in a marital relationship through the facilitation of interaction (Jacob & Leonard 1988).

The availability theory suggests that the greater the availability of alcohol or other psychoactive substances, the greater the prevalence and severity of substance use problems in society. According to Ghodse (1995), the availability of the drug is a prerequisite for misuse and dependence and the rapid transport system of the modern world ensures that drugs or alcohol are obtainable everywhere. Other factors such as relative cost, social pressures, legal sanctions and marketing practices may have a significant influence in the initiation or maintenance of addiction.

Table 6.1 Multifaceted models of addiction.

	Moral	Disease	Neuropharmacological/ genetic	Psychological	Sociological	Bio-psychosocial
Aetiology	Deviated from religious and sociocultural norms	Biological factors, possibly genetic	Pharmacological effects of drugs on the brain Genetic predisposition	Conflict in psychosexual development Learned problem behaviours Reinforcements	Environmental and social factors	Recognises that there are multiple pathways to addiction
Intervention strategies	Control of behaviour: spiritual guidance or punishment	Abstinence is the only option	Pharmacological interventions	Cognitive-behavioural interventions	Improved social functioning	Holistic approach Pharmacological and non-pharmacological interventions
Pros of model	Responsibility for change lies with the user	Not blaming or punitive Adoption of sick role	Not blaming or punitive	Not blaming or punitive	Easily integrated into other models	Multifaceted Dealing with complex behaviours
Cons of model	Victim blaming Punitive approach	Individual not responsible for disease	Individual not responsible for disease	Mechanistic approach Ignores social/ environmental factors	Implies change of social situation is sufficient	

The cultural model recognizes that the influence of culture is a strong determinant of whether or not individuals fall prey to certain addictions. Cultural and religious attitudes have been considered to be a defensive shield against alcohol and drug addiction and in some cases legitimise the use of psychoactive substances. Social rules and etiquette in some cultures tend to encourage individuals to view alcohol as a social lubricant and to promote moderate or controlled drinking. Both ethnicity and religious values have a strong influence on the nature and pattern of drug-taking and drinking behaviour (Oyefeso *et al.* 2000). However, drug-taking and drinking patterns may alter as a result of immigration and social and economic constraints. Other sociocultural factors that may have an influence on drug and alcohol use and misuse include gender, age, occupation, social class, ethnocultural background, subculture, alienated groups, family dysfunction and religious affiliation.

Bio-psychosocial theory

There have been several attempts to amalgamate the biological, psychological and sociological theories of addiction into an integrated conceptual framework – the bio-psychosocial perspectives (Van Wormer & Davis 2007) The bio-psychosocial model recognises that there are multiple pathways to addiction and that the significance of these individual pathways depends on the individual. Furthermore, the bio-psychosocial model was one of the first models to apply the holistic approach to care and intervention strategies. Even though the focus here is on biological and psychological processes, social factors are also included in this model through learning, perceiving and interpreting the world about us as well as through the person's social relationships and larger cultural environment. The bio-psychosocial 'vulnerability model' of Kumpter *et al.* (1990) includes biological factors (genetic inheritance, physiological differences) and psychosocial and environmental factors (family, community, peer or social pressure). In addition, another component may be added to the bio-psychosocial theory, that is the spiritual dimension (Hammond & Rassool 2006).

A summary of the multifaceted models of addiction is presented in Table 6.1.

Summary of key points

- Theories or models include the moral theory, genetic theory, neuropharmacological theories, psychoanalytical theory, behavioural theories, social learning theory, personality theory, sociocultural theories and bio-psychosocial theory.
- In the moral theory addictive behaviours are seen as a sign of moral weakness, bad character or having a weak will.

- ■ The disease theory of addiction maintained that addiction is a disease that is firmly attributed to the genetic\biological make-up of the individual or behavioural processes, or of some combination of the two.
- ■ The neuropharmacological theories of addiction require an understanding of the pharmacological effects of drugs on the brain. Psychoactive substances have different actions on the brain based on the reward systems.
- ■ The genetic model put forward a genetic predisposition to alcohol or drug addiction.
- ■ Family studies have shown an increased incidence of alcoholism in families.
- ■ The psychoanalytical theory of addiction believes that addiction stems from fixation at psychosexual development or death wishes.
- ■ Behaviour is learned through the process of classical conditioning and operant conditioning.
- ■ In social learning theory, in order to understand the effects of alcohol or drugs, cognitive processes must be considered in relation to other factors.
- ■ In sociological theories addiction is seen as a socially constructed phenomenon.
- ■ In the bio-psychosocial theory genetic inheritance, physiological differences, the family, the community, and peer or social pressure are all considered.

References

Adrian M. (2003) How can sociological theory help our understanding of addictions? *Substance Use and Misuse*, 38(10), 1385–1423.

Adityanjee D. & Murray R.M. (1991) The role of genetic predisposition in alcoholism. In I.B. Glass (ed.) *The International Handbook of Addiction Behaviour*, pp. 41–47. Tavistock/Routledge, London.

Bandura A. (1977) *Social Learning Theory*. Prentice-Hall, Englewood Cliffs.

Barnes G. (1990) Impact of the family on adolescent drinking patterns. In R. Collins, K. Leonard & J. Searles (eds) *Alcohol and the Family: research and clinical perspectives*, pp. 137–161. Guilford Press, New York.

Bierut L.J., Dinwiddie S.H., Begleiter H. *et al.* (1998) Familial transmission of substance dependence: alcohol, marijuana, cocaine, and habitual smoking. A report from the Collaborative Study on the Genetics of Alcoholism. *Archives of General Psychiatry*, 55(11), 982–988.

Collins R. & Marlatt G. (1981) Social modelling as a determinant of drinking behaviour: implications for prevention and treatment. *Addictive Behaviours*, 6, 233–240.

Diaz J. (1996) *How Drugs Influence Behavior: a neurobehavorial approach*. Prentice Hall, New York.

Drummond D.C., Tiffany S.T., Glautier S. & Remington B. (1995) Cue exposure in understanding and treating addictive behaviours. In D.C. Drummond, S.T. Tiffany, S. Glautier & B. Remington (eds) *Addictive Behaviour: cue exposure theory and practice*, pp. 1–17. Wiley, Chichester, UK.

Eysenck H. (1997) Addiction, personality and motivation. *Human Psychopharmacology*, 12, 79–87.

Ghodse A.H. (1995) *Drugs and Addictive Behaviour*. Blackwell Science, Oxford.

Gianoulakis C. (2001) Influence of the endogenous opioid system on high alcohol consumption and genetic predisposition to alcoholism. *Journal of Psychiatry and Neuroscience*, 26(4), 304–318.

Hammond A. & Rassool G.H. (2006) Spiritual and cultural needs: integration in dual diagnosis care. In G.H. Rassool (ed.) *Dual Diagnosis Nursing*, pp. 209–221. Blackwell Publishing, Oxford.

Heath A. (1995) Genetic influences on alcoholism risk: a review of adoption and twin studies. *Alcohol Health and Research World*, 19(3), 166–171.

Heyman G.M. (2009) *Addiction: a disorder of choice*. Harvard University Press, Cambridge, MA.

Institute of Medicine (1996) *Pathways of Addiction*. National Academy Press, Washington, DC.

Jacob T. & Leonard K. (1988) Alcohol–spouse interaction as a function of alcoholism subtype and alcohol consumption interaction. *Journal of Abnormal Psychology*, 97(2), 231–237.

Kumpter K.L., Trunnell E.P. & Whiteside, H.O. (1990) The biopsychosocial model: applications to the addictions field. In R.C. Eng (ed.) *Controversies in the Addictions Field*, Vol. 1, pp. 55–67. Kendall/Hunt Publishing Co., Dubuque, IA.

Leeds J. & Morgenstern J. (1996) Psychoanalytic theories of substance abuse. In F. Rotgers, D.S. Keller & J. Morgenstern (eds) *Treating Substance Abuse: theory and technique*, pp. 68–83. Guilford Press, New York.

Merikangas K.R., Stevens D.E., Fenton B., Stolar M., O'Malley S., Woods S.W. & Risch N. (1998) Co-morbidity and familial aggregation of alcoholism and anxiety disorders. *Psychological Medicine*, 28(4), 773–788.

Merton R. (1971) Social problems and sociological theory. In R. Merton & R. Nisbet (eds) *Contemporary Social Problems*, pp. 697–737. Harcourt Brace Jovanovich, New York.

Miller N.S. (1991) *The Pharmacology of Alcohol and Drugs of Abuse and Addiction*. Springer-Verlag, New York.

Nutt D. (1997) The neurochemistry of addiction. *Human Psychopharmacology*, 12, 53–58.

Nutt D. & Lingford-Hughes A. (2008) Addiction: the clinical interface. *British Journal of Pharmacology*, 154(2), 397–405.

Orford J. (1985) *Excessive Appetites: a psychological view of addictions*. John Wiley & Sons, Chichester, UK.

Oyefeso A., Ghodse H., Keating A., Annan J., Phillips T., Pollard M. & Nash P. (2000) *Drug Treatment Needs of Black and Minority Ethnic residents of the London Borough of Merton*. Addictions Resource Agency for Commissioners (ARAC) Monograph Series on Ethnic Minority Issues. ARAC, London.

Sher K., Walitzer K., Wood P. & Brent E. (1991) Characteristics of children of alcoholics: putative risk factors, substance use and abuse, and psychopathology. *Journal of Abnormal Psychology*, 100(4), 427–448.

Steinglass P. (1987) A systems view of family interaction and psychopathology. In T. Jacob (ed.) *Family Interaction and Psychopathology: theories, methods, and findings*, pp. 25–65. Plenum, New York.

Treece C. & Khantzian E.J. (1986) Psychodynamic factors in the development of drug dependence. *Psychiatric Clinics of North America*, 9(3), 399–412.

Tsuang M.T., Lyons M.J., Eisen S.A. *et al.* (1996) Genetic influences on DSM III-R. Drug abuse and dependence. A study of 3372 pairs of twins. *American Journal of Medical Genetics*, 67(5), 473–477.

Van Wormer K.S. & Davis D.R. (2007) *Addiction Treatment: a strengths perspective*. Thomson Brooks/ Cole, Florence, KY.

Vengeliene V., Bilbao A., Molander A. & Spanagel R. (2008) Neuropharmacology of alcohol addiction. *British Journal of Pharmacology*, 154(2), 299–315.

West R. (2006) *Theory of Addiction*. Blackwell Publishing, Oxford.

7 Models of Care and Change

Contemporary health care systems face considerable challenges in providing quality care as a consequence of the changing pattern and nature of addiction, the expectations of service users and carers, and a greater emphasis on quality and accountability. A 'nursing model' pertains solely to the practice domain of nursing, whereas a 'model of care' describes the delivery of health care within the broader context of the health system (Davidson *et al.* 2006). *Models of Care for Treatment of Adult Drug Misusers* or *MoCDM* (NTA 2002) sets out a national framework, in England, for the commissioning of adult treatment for drug misuse to meet the needs of diverse local populations. *Models of Care for Alcohol Misusers* or *MoCAM* (NTA 2007) is based on all the key foundations laid down in the document *MoCDM* (NTA 2002). The 'Models of Care' framework for drug and alcohol misusers advocates a whole system approach to meeting the multiple needs of substance misusers through the development of local systems that integrate drug and alcohol treatment services with other generic health, social and criminal justice services, including throughcare and aftercare.

Models of care: drugs

MoCDM and *MoCDM Updated* (NTA 2002, 2006) include the key tenets of care planning and coordination of care and the development of integrated care pathways. In addition, there are definitions of the full range of treatment interventions in the context of local treatment systems, with a particular focus on reducing the risk of immediate death due to overdoses and risks of morbidity and mortality due to blood-borne viruses and other infections. This may include the provision of interventions to reduce drug-related harm such as increasing the availability of clean injecting equipment, interventions to encourage drug injectors not to share injecting equipment, to use ingestion methods as an alternative to injecting, and to attract drug users into oral substitute treatment when appropriate.

MoCDM (NTA 2002) introduced a four tiers' system of models of care. A summary of the key points is presented in Table 7.1. Tier 1 services are generic (non-substance misuse specific) services, which include the provision of their own services plus, as a minimum, screening and referral to local drug and alcohol treatment services in tiers 2 and 3. The aim of the treatment in tier 2 is to engage substance abusers in drug treatment and reduce drug-related harm. This tier includes services such as needle exchange, drug and alcohol advice and information services, low-threshold prescribing programmes, and ad hoc support not delivered in the context of a care plan.

Tier 3 services are specialist services provided solely for drug and alcohol misusers in structured programmes of care. They require that drug and alcohol misusers receive a drug assessment and have a care plan and a whole gamut of pharmacotherapy and psychosocial interventions. Tier 3 services and mental health services should work closely together to meet the needs of drug misusers with dual diagnosis. Tier 4 services are aimed at individuals with complex needs and include in-patient drug and alcohol units, residential rehabilitation units and crisis intervention centres.

Models of care: alcohol

MoCAM identifies four main categories of alcohol misusers who may benefit from some kind of intervention or treatment: hazardous drinkers, harmful drinkers, moderately dependent drinkers and severely dependent drinkers. The key points of the four-tiered framework are presented in Table 7.2.

Tier 1 interventions include provision of information on sensible drinking, simple brief interventions to reduce alcohol-related harm and referral of those with alcohol dependence. Tier 2 interventions include provision of alcohol-specific advice, information and support, extended brief interventions, and assessment and referral of those with more serious alcohol-related problems for care-planned treatment. Tier 3 interventions include provision of community-based specialised alcohol misuse assessment that is care coordinated and planned. Tier 4 interventions include provision of residential, specialised alcohol treatments that are care planned and coordinated to ensure continuity of care and aftercare.

Table 7.1   Models of care: drugs.

Tier	Settings	Professionals	Intervention strategies
1	Primary health care services Acute hospitals, e.g. A&E departments Psychiatric services Social services departments Homelessness services Antenatal clinics General hospital wards Police settings, e.g. custody cells Probation services Prison service Education and vocational services Occupational health services Hepatology services	Primary care General medical services Social workers Community pharmacists Probation officers Housing officers Homeless persons units	Drug and alcohol screening Referral to alcohol and drug services Assessment Information to reduce drug-related harm Liaison with drug and alcohol services General medical care Housing support Hepatitis B vaccination
2	Drug advice and information centres Drop-in services Pharmacy Outreach services Self-referrals Referral from a variety of other sources	Specialist drug and alcohol workers Specialist social workers	Drug and alcohol screening and assessment Care planning and management Criminal justice screening and referral Motivation and brief interventions Drug and alcohol information services Needle exchange Ad hoc support (no care planning) Social work advice Childcare/parenting assessment Assessment of social care needs Low-threshold prescribing programme Outreach work

Table 7.1 *Continued*

Tier	Settings	Professionals	Intervention strategies
3	Community-based specialist drug and alcohol services Structured community-based services for stimulant users, young people, black and minority ethnic groups, women, HIV (Human Immune Deficiency Syndrome) and AIDS (acquired immune deficiency syndrome), dual diagnosis Self-referrals Referral from a variety of sources	Specialist drug and alcohol workers Dual diagnosis workers Specialist social workers	Drug assessment Care plan Care coordinator Shared care prescribing Testing order drug treatment Cognitive-behavioural therapy Motivational interventions Counselling Methadone maintenance programmes Community detoxification Day care Aftercare programme
4a	In-patient drug and alcohol detoxification services Drug and alcohol residential rehabilitation units Residential drug crisis intervention centres Referral from tiers 2 or 3 services	Drug and alcohol specialist workers Counsellors/therapists Specialist liaison services to tiers 1–4a services	Provision of holistic care: physical, psychological, social and spiritual care Pharmacotherapy Psychological interventions Social interventions Educational interventions
4b	Non-substance misuse specific	Specialist liver disease units HIV clinics and genitourinary clinics Eating disorders units Forensic services Personality disorder units Terminal care services	

Source: adapted from NTA (National Treatment Agency) (2002) *Models of Care for Treatment of Adult Drug Misusers. Parts 1 and 2*. NTA Publications, London. NTA (National Treatment Agency) (2006) *Models of Care for Treatment of Adult Drug Misusers Updated*. NTA Publications, London.

Transtheoretical model of change

The transtheoretical model (Prochaska *et al.* 1992; Prochaska & Velicer 1997) is an integrative model of behaviour change that involves emotions, cognition and behaviour. In this model, behavioural change is viewed as a process with

Table 7.2 Models of care: alcohol.

Tier	Settings	Specialist settings	Intervention strategies
1	Primary health care services Acute hospitals, e.g. A&E departments Psychiatric services Social services departments Homelessness services Antenatal clinics General hospital wards Police settings, e.g. custody cells Probation services Prison service Education and vocational services Occupational health services	Specialist liver disease units Specialist psychiatric wards Forensic units Residential provision for the homeless Domestic abuse services	Interventions include the identification of hazardous, harmful and dependent drinkers Information on sensible drinking Simple brief interventions to reduce alcohol-related harm Referral of those with alcohol dependence or harm for more intensive interventions
2	Primary health care services Acute hospitals, e.g. A&E departments Psychiatric services Social services departments Homelessness services Antenatal clinics General hospital wards Police settings, e.g. custody cells Probation services Prison service Education and vocational services Occupational health services	Alcohol services	Alcohol-specific information, advice and support Extended brief interventions and brief treatment to reduce alcohol-related harm Alcohol-specific assessment and referral of those requiring more structured alcohol treatment Partnership or shared care with staff from tiers 3 and 4 Provision for or joint care of individuals attending other services provided in tier 1 Interventions Mutual aid groups, e.g. Alcoholics Anonymous Triage assessment, which may be provided as part of locally agreed arrangements

Table 7.2 *Continued*

Tier	Settings	Specialist settings	Intervention strategies
3	Primary care settings (shared care schemes) GP-led prescribing services The work in community settings can be delivered by statutory, voluntary or independent services providing care-planned, structured alcohol treatment	Community-based, structured, care-planned alcohol treatment	Comprehensive substance misuse assessment Care planning Case management Community detoxification Prescribing interventions to reduce risk of relapse Psychosocial therapies and support Interventions to address coexisting conditions Day programmes Liaison services, e.g. for acute medical and psychiatric health services (such as pregnancy, mental health or hepatitis services) Social care services (such as child care and housing services) and other generic services
4	In-patient provision in the context of general psychiatric wards Hospital services for pregnancy, liver problems, etc. with specialised alcohol liaison support	Alcohol specialist in-patient treatment and residential rehabilitation	Comprehensive substance misuse assessment Care planning and review Prescribing interventions Alcohol detoxification Prescribing interventions to reduce risk of relapse Psychosocial therapies and support Provision of information, advice and training, and shared care, to others

Source: adapted from NTA (National Treatment Agency) (2006) *Models of Care for Treatment of Adult Drug Misusers Updated*. NTA Publications, London.

individuals at various levels of motivation or stages for 'readiness' to change. As individuals will be at different stages in this process of change, intervention strategies should match their particular stage. Proponents of the model have argued that interventions that are tailored to a particular stage of change improve the effectiveness of the individual to change (Prochaska & Velicer 1997). This model of change is a circular rather than a linear model. The individual may go through several cycles of contemplation, action and relapse before either reaching maintenance, termination or exiting the system without remaining free from substance misuse. The stages of change model considers relapse to be normal. Despite its popularity in the addiction and health promotion fields, there are inherent problems with the model, many of which have been well articulated (Sutton 2001; Littell & Girvin 2002).

Stages of change

The model construes change as a process involving progress through a series of six stages: pre-contemplation, contemplation, preparation, action, maintenance and termination or relapse (Figure 7.1):

1 *Pre-contemplation:* In this stage, individuals have no insight of the problem or are unaware of the problem and have no intention of changing.
2 *Contemplation:* Individuals are seriously contemplating a change in behaviour. They are aware of the pros and the cons of behavioural change.
3 *Preparation:* At the preparation stage, an individual recognises the problem and intends to change the behaviour.
4 *Action:* Action is the stage in which people have made specific overt changes in their lifestyle and behaviour.
5 *Maintenance:* At this stage, individuals continue with desirable and acceptable behaviours. They are working to prevent relapse and consolidate gains secured during the action phase.
6 *Termination or relapse:* In the termination phase, individuals have gained adequate self-efficacy to eliminate the risk of lapse or relapse. Most substance misusers experience relapse on the journey to permanent cessation or stable reduction of high-risk behaviours.

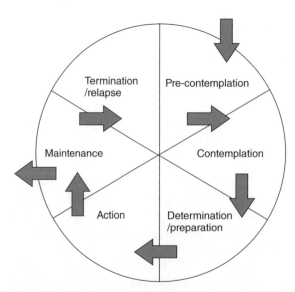

Figure 7.1 A model of the Process of Change (Prochaska and DiClemente, 1986).

The stage of change model is of practical value when selecting appropriate interventions. By identifying an individual position in the change process, intervention strategies such as support, advice, brief interventions and counselling can be tailored to match an individual's readiness to change (see Rassool 2009a).

Nursing model

It is through the therapeutic process that nurses form relationships with their patients, assessing their needs, making hypotheses, planning goals of intervention, implementing care and evaluating the care provided. A nursing model is a 'collection of ideas, knowledge and values about nursing which determines the way nurses, as individuals and groups, work with their patients or clients' (Wright 1990). According to Aggleton and Chalmers (2000) nursing models have a number of components, which include:

■ The nature of planning and goal setting.
■ The focus of intervention during implementation of the care plan.
■ The nature of evaluation.
■ The role of the nurse.

Nursing models give a systematic direction to nursing care. The most popular and widely used model in the UK and elsewhere is the Roper, Logan and Tierney (1996) model in adult nursing. In psychiatric nursing, the tidal model (Barker & Buchanan-Barker 2005), Orem self-care deficit theory (Orem 2001) or Peplau's interpersonal relations model (Peplau 1991) are frequently used. Within these frameworks or models is the nursing process, which includes the processes of assessment, planning, implementation and evaluation.

Assessment

Assessment is one of the stages in the systematic approach to nursing care and interventions. Nursing assessment focuses on gathering information on the physiological, psychological, sociological and spiritual needs of the patient. The purposes of assessment are to:

■ Build a rapport with the patient.
■ Gather information for the planning of care.
■ Intervene in urgent medical and psychological problems.
■ Provide feedback to patients.
■ Evaluate the effectiveness of clinical practice.

Assessment by nurses is an ongoing process and there is a need to appreciate that the care needs of the patient are constantly changing with differing physical or

Table 7.3 Guide to effective assessment.

▨ Introduce yourself
▨ Be courteous
▨ Be aware of the immediate needs of the patient
▨ Intervene appropriately to the patient's urgent needs
▨ Use non-verbal communication
▨ Use empathy and not sympathy
▨ Use opened and closed questions
▨ Listen
▨ Clarify
▨ Reflect
▨ Paraphrase
▨ Summarise
▨ Make notes

psychosocial needs. A guide to effective assessment is presented in Table 7.3. The assessment is then documented on paper or electronic records, which can be accessed by all members of the health care team.

Engagement is concerned with the development and maintenance of a therapeutic relationship between the nurse and the patient. Confrontational and judgmental approaches may exacerbate the potential for patients to disengage with nursing interventions. The process of assessment can be enhanced by the style of interaction, which should be non-confrontational, empathic and respectful of the client's subjective experiences of substance misuse. Issues of alcohol and drug misuse are not addressed directly until the end of the engagement process, when a working alliance has developed (Rassool 2009b).

Key principles in care planning

The planning phase of patient needs involves the development of a care plan and is a key component of the structured nursing process. The care planning process is a method for setting goals based on the needs identified during the assessment phases. In addition, the care plan is also: (i) a tool to monitor any changes in the patient's needs; (ii) a guide for the basis for continuity of care; (iii) it shows accountability; and (iv) it is a legal document. However, the effectiveness of the care plan is based on the engagement of the patient throughout the assessment and care planning process and being actively involved in the formulation of the care plan. Every patient should have a documented care plan that is individualised to the patient's needs, develops with the patient and significant others, reflects evidence-based practice and nursing interventions, and provides for continuity of aftercare.

A care plan should have SMART (specific, measurable, achievable, realistic, time-limited) goals or objectives. The goals must be stated in terms of patient achievement and each goal must state a target date for evaluation. Key areas of risk behaviours, management of risk and emergency planning should be made explicit in the care plan. Each goal must be accompanied by an evidence-based nursing intervention. The care plan should be monitored, reviewed and evaluated at regular intervals. Reviewing a care plan provides a framework within which the nurse and the patient can decide whether needs have been met or goals have been achieved. The key principles in care planning are presented in Tables 7.4 and 7.5.

Implementing the care plan

This is the third stage of the process of nursing and involved the provision of nursing interventions. The skills of nursing interventions include interpersonal, cognitive and technical skills.

Table 7.4 Key principles in care planning.

Client-centred approach	▪ Client-directed ▪ Holistic needs of client ▪ Involved in decision making about the components of the care plan and how it will be delivered
Diversity	▪ Reflect the patient's cultural and ethnic background, gender and sexuality
Goals	▪ Need to reflect the outcome of the assessment ▪ Based on philosophy of care ▪ SMART – specific, measurable, achievable, realistic and time-bound ▪ Taking account of individual's current state and motivation ▪ Short-term and long-term goals
Nursing intervention strategies	▪ Type of interventions: physical, pharmacological and psychosocial
Risk management	▪ Identification of risk factors as per assessment ▪ Risk management and contingency plan
Communication and liaison	▪ Sharing of information in line with service policies on confidentiality and the sharing of information
Nurse as key worker	▪ Developing, implementing and evaluating a care plan ▪ Deliver heath and psychosocial interventions
Promoting and enhancing engagement	▪ Where an individual has been difficult to engage in treatment and rehabilitation, the plan should identify a plan for promoting and enhancing their engagement
Monitor	▪ Monitor plan and changes in client's needs
Review	▪ Identity their review date

Source: adapted from Rassool G.H. (2009b) *Alcohol and Drug Misuse. A handbook for student and health professionals.* Routledge, Oxford. Reproduced with kind permission of Taylor & Francis.

Table 7.5 Effective care planning.

Key areas of care planning	Examples
Establish the problems	Problems related to physical or psychosocial needs
Establish the risks and priorities	Risk of suicide, overdose, etc.
	Emergency interventions
Monitor vital signs	Can the patient breath adequately?
Is the patient in pain? Discomfort?	Physical and/or psychological
Can the patient maintain a safe environment?	Alcohol intoxication and aggressive or violent behaviours
Non-compliance with nursing interventions and medical advice	

Evaluating the care plan

For many patients, a change in health care needs or situation, or a crisis, provides an opportunity for a review of the care plan. However, a care plan with its goals and associated nursing interventions should be monitored and reviewed when necessary. The evaluation should be recorded and a general statement included about the achievement of goal(s), and the care plan is amended if circumstances have changed.

Summary of key points

■ *Models of Care for Treatment of Adult Drug Misusers (MoCDM)* sets out a national framework, in England, for the commissioning of adult treatment for drug misuse to meet the needs of diverse local populations and to improve the quality and effectiveness of drug treatment.

■ *Models of Care for Alcohol Misusers (MoCAM)* sets a national framework for England for the development of structured treatment and of integrated care pathways for those who misuse alcohol.

■ The transtheoretical model construes change as a process involving progress through a series of six stages: pre-contemplation, contemplation, preparation, action, maintenance and termination or relapse.

■ Assessment, care planning and care coordination are key components of an integrated nursing intervention.

■ The first step in care planning is accurate and comprehensive assessment.

■ Care planning provides a 'road map' of the patient's needs and goals.

■ The care planning process is a method for setting goals based on the needs identified by an assessment, and planning interventions to meet those goals with the patient.

■ A care plan is a structured and task-oriented plan of action between the patient and the nurse (key worker).

■ The planning of interventions is based upon the needs or goals identified in the care planning process.

References

Aggleton P. & Chalmers H. (2000) *Nursing Models and Nursing Practice*, 2nd edn. Macmillan, London.

Barker, P. & Buchanan-Barker P. (2005) *The Tidal Model: a guide for mental health professionals.* Brunner-Routledge, London.

Davidson P., Halcomb E., Hickman L., Phillips J. & Graham B. (2006) Beyond the rhetoric: what do we mean by a 'model of care'? *Australian Journal of Advanced Nursing*, 23(3), 47–55.

Littell J.H. & Girvin H. (2002) Stages of change. A critique. *Behavior Modification*, 26(2), 223–273.

NTA (National Treatment Agency) (2002) *Models of Care for Treatment of Adult Drug Misusers. Parts 1 and 2.* NTA Publications, London.

NTA (National Treatment Agency) (2006) *Models of Care for Treatment of Adult Drug Misusers Updated*. NTA Publications, London.

NTA (National Treatment Agency) (2007) *Models of Care for Alcohol Misusers.* Department of Health, London.

Orem D.E. (2001) *Nursing: concepts of practice*, 6th edn. Mosby, London.

Peplau H.E. (1991) *Interpersonal Relations in Nursing: a conceptual framework of reference for psychodynamic nursing.* Springer Publishing, New York.

Prochaska J.O. and DiClemente C.C. (1986) Towards a comprehensive model of change, in W.R. Miller and N. Heather (eds.) *Treating addictive behaviors: processes of change*, New York: Plenum.

Prochaska J.O., DiClemente C.C. & Norcross J.C. (1992) In search of how people change. *American Psychologist*, 47(9), 1102–1114.

Prochaska J.O. & Velicer W.K. (1997) The trans-theoretical model of health behaviour change. *American Journal of Health Promotion*, 12(1), 38–48.

Rassool G.H. (2009a) Strategies in helping people to change. In G.H. Rassool *Alcohol and Drug Misuse. A handbook for student and health professionals*, pp. 297–308. Routledge, Oxford.

Rassool G.H. (2009b) *Alcohol and Drug Misuse. A handbook for student and health professionals.* Routledge, Oxford.

Roper N., Logan W.W. & Tierney A.J. (1996) *The Elements of Nursing: a model for nursing based on a model for living*, 4th edn. Churchill Livingstone, London.

Sutton S. (2001) Back to the drawing board? A review of applications of the transtheoretical model to substance use. *Addiction*, 96(1), 175–186.

Wright S.G. (1990) *Building and Using a Model for Nursing*, 2nd edn. Edward Arnold, London.

8 Alcohol

Alcohol is part of the social and cultural fabric and is actively promoted in many cultural, social and religious circumstances. However, alcohol is not generally perceived as a psychoactive substance with addictive potential resulting in physical, psychological, social, economic and legal consequences. Public health problems associated with alcohol consumption have reached alarming proportions, and alcohol has become one of the most important risks to health globally (WHO 2004).

Around 2 billion people worldwide consume alcoholic beverages and over 76 million people have alcohol use disorders (WHO 2007). From a public health perspective, the global burden related to alcohol consumption, both in terms of morbidity and mortality, is substantial in most parts of the world. The World

Health Organization (WHO 2007) estimates that harmful use of alcohol causes about 2.3 million premature deaths per year worldwide and is responsible for 4.4% of the global burden of disease.

In Europe, alcohol is public health enemy number 3, behind only tobacco and high blood pressure, and ahead of obesity, lack of exercise and illicit drugs. The UK is one of the top bingeing nations in Western Europe, binge drinking per person 28 times per year on average – about once every 13 days. UK adolescents are also the third worst binge drinkers in the European Union, with more than a quarter of 15–16 year olds binge drinking three or more times in the last month (Anderson & Baumberg 2007). An overview of alcohol and its effects are presented in Table 8.1.

What is a unit of alcohol?

One unit of alcohol = half a pint of ordinary strength beer, lager or cider (3–4% alcohol by volume (ABV)) = a small pub measure of spirits (40% ABV) = a standard pub measure (50 ml) of fortified wine (sherry or port) (20% ABV) = a small glass of ordinary strength wine (12% ABV) = a standard pub measure of spirits (40% ABV).

The exact number of units in a particular drink can be calculated by multiplying the volume of the drink (number of millilitres) by the %ABV and dividing by 1000:

■ For example, the number of units in 500 ml of a strong beer with a 6% ABV = 500 × 6.0 divided by 1000 = 3 units.

Another way of calculating units is as follows: the %ABV of a drink equals the number of units in 1 litre of that drink:

■ For example, strong beer with a 6% ABV has 6 units in 1 litre. If you drink half a litre (500 ml) – just under a pint – then you have had 3 units.

Health consequences of alcohol use

The trend in the rate of alcohol-related deaths is now levelling out following rapid increases since the early 1990s according to the Office for National Statistics (ONS 2009). The data on alcohol-related deaths in the UK for 2007 show that there were 8724 alcohol-related deaths in 2007, lower than in 2006. In 2007, the alcohol-related death rate for all persons was 13.3 per 100 000 population, compared with 6.9 per 100 000 in 1991. Alcohol-related death rates among males have been consistently higher than rates for females, although trends demonstrate a broadly similar pattern across different age groups. Since 1991, the highest death rates for men and women have occurred in those aged 55–74 years. In contrast, the lowest rates have been in men and women aged 15–34 (ONS 2009). The

Table 8.1 Characteristics of alcohol.

Street names	■ Booze, nip, tipple, bevy, etc. ■ Found in beer, lager, alcopops, cider, wine, spirits, etc.
Legal status	■ Supply of alcohol to anyone under the age of 5 is illegal unless medically indicated ■ Over the age of 5, young people may legally drink (but not purchase) alcohol, though not on licensed premises, and a parent or carer may commit an offence if a child in their care becomes drunk ■ Young people aged 16 and over may purchase beer, cider and sherry in licensed premises for consumption with a table meal. Otherwise, the sale of alcohol to under 18 year olds is forbidden ■ It is an offence to be drunk in a public place, and in pubs, or to drive while unfit through drink ■ The Confiscation of Alcohol (Young Persons) Act 1997 permits police to confiscate alcohol in public places from people under the age of 19 if they judge that it might otherwise lead to a nuisance or to disturbance being committed
Therapeutic use	■ As an antiseptic
Recommended limit	■ The government's recommendations on daily consumption are: less than 3–4 units a day for men, and 2–3 units a day for women
Short-term effects	■ Effects vary according to the strength of the drink, and the person's physical size and mood ■ Feeling of relaxation and euphoria ■ Experience less inhibition ■ Speech can become slurred, coordination is affected and emotions heightened ■ Poor judgment ■ Insomnia ■ Hangover
Long-term effects	■ Overdose can lead to loss of consciousness and alcoholic poisoning, which can be fatal ■ Physical dependence can occur ■ Menstrual disorders ■ Fertility problems ■ Fetal alcohol syndrome ■ Physical problems ■ Psychological problems ■ Social problems

prevalence of alcohol dependence overall equates to 1.1 million people with alcohol dependence nationally. Men are more likely to drink normal strength beer, lager and cider and less likely to drink strong beer, lager and cider and women are more likely to drink wine and less likely to drink strong beer, lager and cider and alcopops (ONS 2006).

Alcohol misuse is associated with a wide range of problems, including cancer, heart disease, offending behaviours, social exclusion, domestic violence, suicide and deliberate self-harm, child abuse, child neglect, mental health problems that coexist with alcohol misuse, and homelessness. Rising levels of consumption are most pronounced in women and young people, with the latter more prone to heavy binge drinking. UK adults and adolescents are among the worst binge drinkers in Europe according to an Institute of Alcohol Studies report (Anderson 2007). Men are more likely to be admitted with alcoholic liver disease than women and twice as many men as women are admitted with this diagnosis. Most of the alcohol-related deaths are caused by cirrhosis and chronic liver disease, but many also result from accidental alcohol poisoning or other problems. Alcohol misuse imposes a greater burden on the criminal justice system than both the health service and social work services. A summary of the problems associated with harmful drinking is presented in Table 8.2.

Wernicke's encephalopathy is caused by alcohol and thiamine (vitamin B) deficiency and is characterised by unsteady gait (ataxia), involuntary, jerky eye movements or paralysis of the muscles moving the eyes, drowsiness and confusion. If treatment with high doses of thiamine is carried out in time most symptoms should be reversed in a few hours. If Wernicke's encephalopathy is untreated or is not treated soon enough, Korsakoff's psychosis may follow.

Table 8.2 Problems associated with alcohol intoxication.

Physical	Psychological	Social
Accidents	Anger	Absenteeism
Acute alcohol poisoning	Anxiety	Aggression
Cardiac arrhythmia	Amnesia	Assault
Failure to take prescribed medications	Attempted suicide	Burglary
Fetal damage	Depression	Child neglect/abuse
Gastritis	Impaired relationships	Domestic violence
Gout	Insomnia	Drinking and driving
Hepatitis	Suicide	Family arguments
HIV (through sexual behaviour)		Football hooliganism
Impotence		Homicide
Pancreatitis		Public drunkenness
Stroke		Theft
		Unsafe sex
		Unwanted pregnancy

Source: adapted from Royal College of Psychiatrists (1986) *Alcohol: our favourite drug.* Tavistock Publications, London.

Korsakoff's psychosis differs from most dementias, where there is often damage to a large area of the cortex (the outer part of the brain). The major symptoms of Korsakoff's syndrome are: anterograde and retrograde amnesia, or severe memory loss; confabulation (invented events to fill gaps in memory); apathy; and talkative behaviour in some cases and repetitive behaviour in others. Other problems associated with heavy alcohol consumption include peripheral neuropathies (lack of sensation or pain in the limbs), 'alcohol dementia', and physical, immunological and psychological disorders. There appears to be a strong association between the degree to which an individual is dependent on alcohol and the severity of the problems experienced by the individual and this is independent from the amount of alcohol consumed.

Alcohol withdrawal syndrome

Alcohol dependence involves both physical and psychological dependence. The presence of physical dependence is shown when problem drinkers cease or reduce alcohol consumption. The alcohol withdrawal syndrome is a set of symptoms that individuals have when they suddenly stop drinking alcohol, following continuous and heavy consumption. Some individuals have tremors, seizures and hallucinations, typically occurring within 6–48 hours after the last alcoholic drink. Withdrawals can be mild, moderate or severe (Table 8.3). For most problem

Table 8.3 Alcohol withdrawal symptoms.

Mild to moderate psychological symptoms	Mild to moderate physical symptoms	Severe symptoms
Feeling of shakiness	Headache	A state of confusion and
Feeling of anxiety	Sweating (palms and face)	hallucinations (visual or
Irritable or easily excited	Nausea	tactile): delirium tremens
Emotionally volatile	Vomiting	Clouding of consciousness
Rapid emotional changes	Loss of appetite	Agitation
Depression	Insomnia	Disorientation of time and
Fatigue	Paleness	place
Difficulty with thinking clearly	Rapid heart rate (palpitations)	Paranoid delusions
Bad dreams	Enlarged, dilated pupils	Fear, suspicion and anger
	Skin clammy	Suicidal behaviour
	Abnormal movements	Elevated temperature
	Tremor of hands	Convulsions
	Involuntary movements of the eyelids	Black outs

Source: adapted from Finn D.A. & Crabbe J.C. (1997) Exploring alcohol withdrawal syndrome. *Alcohol Health and Research World*, 21(2), 149–156.

drinkers, alcohol withdrawal will not progress to the severe stage of delirium tremens (confusion and hallucination). When an individual has severe withdrawal symptoms, this can be a life-threatening condition and requires supervision under medical care.

Assessment

Assessment and care planning are a continuing process and a foundation for good clinical practice. It is only one of the stages in the systematic approach to care and interventions. The purposes of assessment are to:

- Gather information for the planning of care and health or social care interventions.
- Intervene in urgent medical and psychological problems.
- Provide feedback for the client on their level of substance misuse.
- Build a rapport with the client.
- Identify the areas that require interventions.

Individuals with alcohol and psychiatric problems have complex or multiple needs which are often difficult to assess comprehensively. Prior to undertaking a comprehensive assessment, there are some observations that may indicate substance misuse and/or mental health problem(s). This may warrant further investigations in the process of assessment. For a detailed description see Rassool and Winnington (2006) and Rassool (2009a).

Initial assessment and screening

The initial assessment or screening is usually carried out in generic settings such as in hospital or primary health care. Screening or initial assessment is a brief process that aims to determine whether an individual has a drug and alcohol problem, health-related problems and risk behaviours (Rassool 2009a). Substance misusers may be present in accident and emergency departments with overdose, self-harm, lost prescriptions, withdrawal seizures, delirium tremens and withdrawal syndrome. Through the assessment process, there is a window of opportunity to provide brief interventions, harm reduction strategies and to motivate substance misusers to move from a pre-contemplation to a contemplation stage of change.

The CAGE questionnaire is the simplest and its four questions could easily be incorporated in the routine assessment process (Table 8.4). Two or more positive responses are said to identify a problem drinker. This short questionnaire concentrates on the consequences rather than on the quantity or frequency of alcohol use.

A number of screening instruments have been introduced to assess alcohol intake and Table 8.5 presents the FAST alcohol screening test.

Table 8.4 The CAGE questionnaire.

▨ Have you ever felt that you should *cut* down your drinking?
▨ Have people *annoyed* you by criticizing your drinking?
▨ Have you ever felt bad or *guilty* about your drinking?
▨ Have you ever had a drink first thing in the morning to steady your nerves, or get rid of a hangover (*eye-opener*)?

Table 8.5 The FAST alcohol screening test.

1 How often do you have eight or more drinks on one occasion?
__ Never __ Less than monthly __ Monthly __ Weekly __ Daily or almost daily

2 How often during the last year have you been unable to remember what happened the night before because you had been drinking?
__ Never __ Less than monthly __ Monthly __ Weekly __ Daily or almost daily

3 How often during the last year have you failed to do what was normally expected of you because of your drinking?
__ Never __ Less than monthly __ Monthly __ Weekly __ Daily or almost daily

4 Has a relative or friend, a doctor or other health worker been concerned about your drinking or suggested you cut down?
__ No __ Yes, but not in the last year __ Yes in the last year

Scoring the FAST test
Score questions 1, 2 and 3 as follows:

▨ Never: 0 points
▨ Less than monthly: 1 point
▨ Monthly: 2 points
▨ Weekly: 3 points
▨ Daily or almost daily: 4 points

Score question 4 as follows:

▨ No: 0 points
▨ Yes, but not in the last year: 2 points
▨ Yes, in the last year: 4 points

The maximum score is 16. A total score of 3 indicates hazardous drinking.

If a person answers 'never' on the first question, he or she is not a hazardous drinker and the remaining questions are not necessary. If a person answers 'weekly' or 'daily or almost daily' on the first question, he or she is considered a hazardous drinker and the rest of the questions are skipped. If a person answers 'monthly' or 'less than monthly' to the first question, the other three questions are needed to complete the screening for hazardous drinking.

Source: Hodgson C.R., Alwyn T., John B., Thom B. & Smith A. (2002) The Fast Alcohol Screening Test. *Alcohol and Alcoholism*, 37(1), 61–66. Reproduced by kind permission of Oxford University Press.

There are other types of assessment including triage assessment and comprehensive assessment. These types of assessment usually take place when substance misusers first have contact with substance misuse services. Alcohol and drug misusers with complex needs require assessments that are comprehensive and multiprofessional to plan effective care and treatment.

Taking an alcohol history

Taking an alcohol history is a detailed assessment of the current presentation of an individual's alcohol drinking pattern of use. Assessing alcohol intake involves asking a patient how many standard drinks they consume on a daily or weekly basis. Ask about the type of alcohol product, its alcohol content and the size of glass used. Ask 'what's the most you have had to drink on any one day in the past month?' Patients tend not to count heavy drinking episodes in their estimate of average weekly consumption, even if these episodes occur frequently. The assessment should then focus on the current level of dependence, risk behaviours, associated problems, source of help, and periods of abstinence and relapse. In order to ascertain the level of dependence, it is important to ask about experiences of withdrawal symptoms or any medical complications. An outline of the taking an alcohol history is shown in Table 8.6.

Testing for current alcohol use

Alcohol can be measured directly in serum, urine and exhaled air. A number of blood tests can be undertaken to assess the presence of alcohol. Essential investigations include liver function tests (LFT) and measurements of gamma-glutamyl transferase (GGT), asparate transaminase (AST) and mean corpuscle volume (MCV). A summary of these special blood tests for drug and alcohol is given in Table 8.7.

Care planning

A care plan is a structured and task-oriented plan of action between the patient and the health professional. The care plan, a written documentation, is based on the identification of needs or goals, strengths and risks identified by the assessment process and is the main focus of intervention strategies. The needs or problems of an alcohol misuser should be incorporated in the overall care plan. The effectiveness of the care plan is based on the engagement of the patient throughout the assessment and care planning process so he or she should be actively involved in the formulation of the plan. Key areas that can be incorporated into a generic care plan with particular consideration of the needs or problems of a problem drinker are presented in Table 8.8.

Table 8.6 Taking an alcohol history.

▦ **Statement of the need/problem**	Consider the individual's concerns, issues, needs or problems
▦ **Current alcohol use**	Type, quantity, frequency
▦ **Pattern of alcohol use**	Details of alcohol taking for past week/month
▦ **Current use of other substances**	Prescribed, illicit or over-the-counter drugs
▦ **Level of dependence**	Any withdrawal symptoms Evidence of increasing tolerance
▦ **Associated problems**	Any medical, psychiatric, social or legal problems
▦ **Risk behaviours**	Source of injecting equipment Sharing of equipment Knowledge about sterilisation and needle-exchange services Sexual behaviour when intoxicated
▦ **Periods of abstinence/relapse**	Duration Were periods of abstinence voluntary or enforced? Reasons for lapse or relapse
▦ **Sources of help**	Social support systems Statutory agencies Local authorities Voluntary agencies Self-help groups
▦ **Coping strategies and strengths**	Previous strategies in coping with the use of alcohol and drugs Achievements, strengths and positive aspects of the individual

Source: Rassool G.H. & Winnington J. (2006) Framework for multidimensional assessment. In G.H. Rassool (ed.) *Dual Diagnosis Nursing*, p. 181. Blackwell Publishing, Oxford.

Table 8.7 Special laboratory tests for alcohol use.

Tests	Observations
Gamma-glutamyl transferase (GGT)	Elevated before liver damage. More likely to have liver damage at higher readings
Liver function test (LFT)	Check liver damage due to alcohol
Full blood count	Mean red blood cells are raised in heavy chronic drinkers
Asparate transaminase (AST)	High levels suggest alcohol-related liver damage
Uric acid	Increase of urates and possibly gout
Haemoglobin	Anaemia due to poor nutrition or vitamin deficiencies

Source: Rassool G.H. & Winnington J. (2006) Framework for multidimensional assessment. In G.H. Rassool (ed.) *Dual Diagnosis Nursing*, p. 181. Blackwell Publishing, Oxford.

Table 8.8 Alcohol: key areas of a care plan.

Needs or problems	Expected outcome	Interventions
Poor physical health	Improvements in daily intake of nutrition	Assessment of daily intake of nutrients Vitamin supplements
Fear of withdrawal symptoms	Prevention of withdrawal symptoms	Health information and advice
Risk behaviour	To eliminate or reduce risk behaviour	Assessment and monitoring Harm reduction
Anxiety	Control of anxiety	Anxiety/stress management
Detoxification	Client will not experience any physical distress and discomfort while undergoing detoxification	To explain the role of medication in facilitating detoxification and overcoming withdrawal

Detoxification and management of withdrawal

Where alcohol causes physical withdrawal syndromes, detoxification is a treatment intervention. Medically assisted detoxification can be delivered both in the community and in-patient settings. Patients with moderate or severe withdrawal may require in-patient detoxification. The main objectives of pharmacological interventions in alcohol withdrawal are the relief of subjective withdrawal symptoms, the prevention and management of more serious complications, and preparation for more structured psychosocial and educational interventions (Rassool 2009a). The alcohol withdrawal syndrome lasts for about 5 days, with the greatest risk of severe withdrawal symptoms in the first 24 to 48 hours.

During the period of detoxification, chlordiazepoxide or diazepam are safe to use and have an anticonvulsant effect that helps to safeguard against epileptic seizures. The principles of nursing care in alcohol detoxification include monitoring of dehydration, blood pressure, dietary intake, orientation to time, place and person, and sleep. The key areas of nursing care are to:

▓ Promote client safety.
▓ Maintain physiological stability during the withdrawal phase.
▓ Meet physical and psychological needs.
▓ Provide appropriate referral and follow-up.

A framework for the nursing management of alcohol withdrawal is presented in Table 8.9.

Patients need a non-stimulating and non-threatening environment, and low lighting at night will help reduce perceptual disturbances. Whilst detoxification can be a very physical process there are a number of psychological elements that

Table 8.9 A nursing framework for alcohol withdrawal.

Needs	Interventions
Environmental stimuli	Nursing in quiet area with only one member of staff in contact
General	Assess level of consciousness
Body temperature	Control body temperature: apply or remove bed clothing when necessary
Blood pressure	Monitor blood pressure
Foods and fluids	Offer fluids every 60 minutes and record fluid intake
Rest and sleep	Allow rest or sleep between monitoring of vital signs
Elimination	Assist to bathroom and record output
Epigastric distress	Deep breathing and relaxation
Withdrawal	Monitor vital signs and amount of withdrawal
Physical comfort/sleep	Change position if necessary
	Institute measures to help patients to sleep
Medication	Monitor patient's response to medication
	Administer vitamins and mineral supplements as prescribed
Reality orientation	Time, place and person
	Assess presence of hallucinations or delusions
Risk behaviour	Assess for suicidal ideation
Positive reinforcement	Reinforce positive elements of the intervention
Visitors	No visitors during supportive care

Source: adapted from Shaw, J.M., Kolesar, G.S., Sellers, E.M., Kaplan, H.L. & Sandor, P. (1981) Development of optimal treatment tactics for alcohol withdrawal. 1. Assessment and effectiveness of supportive care. *Journal of Clinical Psychopharmacology*, 1, 382–387.

nurses are skilled at observing and managing, including hallucinations, delirium, altered mental states, hypervigilance, anxiety, paranoia, depression, tactile hallucinations and high levels of risk (Moore 2006). There is evidence that therapeutic interventions combined with carefully monitored medication are an important factor in the treatment of alcohol withdrawal syndrome (Bennie 1998).

Intervention strategies

Pharmacological interventions

The standard treatment for alcohol misuse may include pharmacotherapy to alleviate withdrawal symptoms followed by psychosocial interventions. For many years, pharmacological interventions were restricted to the treatment of alcohol withdrawal syndrome and to the use of aversive drugs. However, there are only a limited numbers of drugs that can be used to assist problem drinkers. Antabuse (disulfiram) is an efficient intervention and is used for motivated problem drinkers whose goals are abstinence but the low rate of compliance has made Antabuse

Table 8.10 Characteristics of drugs used in alcohol treatment.

	Naltrexone	Acamprosate	Disulfiram
Definition	Opioid antagonist	Partial co-agonist	Alcohol sensitisation
Dosage	Initial dose: 25 mg/ day for 2 days Maintenance dose: 50 mg/day	Dose: patient ≥60 kg: 1998 mg/day patient <60 kg: 999 mg/day	Initial dose: 500 mg/ day for 14 days Maintenance dose: 125–250 mg/day
Contraindications	Cirrhosis, hepatic insufficiency, opioid dependence, pregnancy	Hepatic insufficiency, pregnancy	Cirrhosis, hepatic insufficiency, epilepsy
Adverse effects	Nausea, vomiting, headache, loss of weight	Headache, diarrhoea, rash, nausea	Rash, sexual dysfunction, acne, fatigue, metallic taste in the mouth
Recommendations	Monitoring of hepatic function	Monitoring of hepatic function Insist on correct taking of medications	Monitoring of hepatic function. Introduction only after an abstinence period of 24–48 hours

intervention less effective. In the last decade, naltrexone and acamprosate have been proposed for the treatment of alcohol dependence syndrome. Several studies have indicated that acamprosate reduces the craving for alcohol and enhances abstinence. Acamprosate's effect is dose dependent and it has a few minor side effects. In addition, there are recent reports documenting that naltrexone and acamprosate are more effective than placebo in the treatment of alcohol disorders (Garbutt *et al*. 1999). The characteristics of drugs used in alcohol treatment are presented in Table 8.10.

Pharmacotherapy is also used in relapse prevention. Disulfiram taken under supervision is an effective component of relapse prevention strategies (Heather *et al*. 2006). Anti-craving medications such as naltrexone and acamprosate may also be used as part of psychosocial interventions, including relapse prevention.

Vitamin deficiency in alcoholism is common and causes Wernicke's encephalopathy and is most frequently seen in heavy drinkers with a poor diet. The Royal College of Physicians (2001) has recommended 200 mg four times a day of oral thiamine and strong vitamin B tablets (30 mg/day) as the treatment of choice for the duration of detoxification. Both supplements could be continued if there is evidence of cognitive impairment (thiamine 50 mg four times a day) or poor diet (vitamin B 30 mg/day).

Brief interventions

Brief intervention, which can be conducted in general health care settings, can help patients reduce the risk of developing alcohol-related problems or hazardous alcohol use. Brief interventions can also be used to encourage those with more serious dependence to accept more intensive treatment within the primary care setting, or referral to specialised alcohol and drug services (WHO 2005). Brief interventions aim to motivate those at risk to change their alcohol (or drug) use behaviour (Babor & Higgins-Biddle 2001). The aim of the intervention is to help the patient understand that their alcohol drinking is putting them at risk and to encourage them to reduce (moderate) their intake rather than abstinence. Brief interventions comprise a single brief advice session or several short (15–30 minutes) counselling sessions and are designed to be conducted by non-specialist or generic health care professionals.

The acronym 'FRAMES' summarises the elements of effective brief interventions (Bien *et al.* 1993): feedback, responsibility, advice, menu, empathy and self-efficacy. Brief interventions delivered in a supportive, non-judgmental manner,

Table 8.11 Elements of effective brief interventions.

Acronym	Elements	Counselling responses
F: feedback	Feedback of personal risk or impairment	'Your difficulty in getting to work on time may be related to your alcohol or drug use' Sharing the results of assessments such as cognitive testing and liver function tests
R: responsibility	Emphasis on personal responsibility for change	'It is your responsibility to make a decision about stopping substance misuse for the next 2 weeks'
A: advice	Clear advice to change	'It is recommended that you stop drinking or drug use for the next 2 weeks, to see if that makes a difference'
M: menu	Menu of alternative change options	'If you cannot reduce or stop your substance misuse, other options can be considered such as AA or NA or referral to specialist services'
E: empathy	Therapeutic empathy as a counselling style	'I understand that this will be difficult for you because you feel alcohol helps you to unwind after a stressful working day'
S: self-efficacy	Enhancement of patient self-efficacy or optimism	'Considering how difficult you find this, I am confident that you have the abilities or strengths to consider changing your behaviour'

Source: adapted from Castro L.A. & Baltieri D.A. (2004) The pharmacologic treatment of the alcohol dependence. *Revista Brasileira de Psiquiatria*, 26, 11.

rather than in the more traditional confrontational style, are associated with better outcomes. Table 8.11 presents the elements of effective brief interventions.

The National Institute for Health and Clinical Excellence (NICE) 2007 guideline on psychosocial interventions recommends that opportunistic brief interventions should:

■ Normally consist of two sessions each lasting 10–45 minutes.
■ Explore ambivalence about drug use and possible treatment, with the aim of increasing motivation to change behaviour.
■ Provide non-judgmental feedback.

In addition, NICE recommended that service providers should routinely provide people who misuse alcohol with information about self-help groups based on 12-step principles such as Alcohol Anonymous.

There is strong evidence for the effectiveness of brief interventions, in a variety of settings, in reducing alcohol consumption among hazardous and harmful drinkers to low-risk levels (NTA 2006). This type of intervention has been found to be more effective than no treatment and is often more effective than intensive interventions (Mattick & Jarvis 1993; WHO Brief Intervention Study Group 1996). However, it is important to note that using a self-help manual is better than minimal advice alone and that the provision of a brief intervention is preferable to no therapeutic intervention (Heather 1998). In summary, brief interventions have been found effective for helping harmful or hazardous drinkers to reduce or stop drinking and for motivating moderate or severe alcohol-dependent users to enter long-term alcohol treatment.

Other psychosocial interventions

The goals of psychosocial interventions are to complement pharmacological interventions (for example, in detoxification or relapse prevention) and to enable clients to regain stability and a healthier lifestyle. Motivational interviewing, drawing heavily on basic counselling skills, is the preliminary psychological intervention in specialist settings for patients with moderate or severe alcohol dependence who are not willing to change their risk behaviour. Motivational interviewing increases the effectiveness of more extensive psychological treatment (Heather *et al.* 2006). For more information see Rassool (2009b).

Cognitive-behavioural approaches have been found to be effective in reducing or stopping alcohol use. The aims are to teach individuals how to control their responses to their environment through improving social, coping and problem-solving skills (Teesson *et al.* 2002). In treatment for alcohol dependence, the goal of cognitive-behavioural therapy is to teach the person to recognise situations in which they are most likely to drink, avoid these circumstances if possible, and to cope with other problems and behaviours that may lead to their alcohol misuse.

Cognitive-behaviour therapy has been shown to be most effective when compared with having no other treatment at all (NIDA 2005); however, when compared with other treatment approaches, studies have had mixed results – some show cognitive-behaviour therapy to be more effective while others show it to be of equal effectiveness to other treatments.

One form of cognitive-behavioural therapy is the community reinforcement approach, which consists of a broad range of treatments aiming to alter the service user's social environment (including the family and vocational environment) so that abstinence is rewarded and intoxication unrewarded (Heather *et al.* 2006). Social behaviour and network therapy can also be used with service users in modifying and maintaining changes in alcohol consumption. The basic premise is to enable clients to develop positive social networks (Copello *et al.* 2002). Marital therapy, based on the cognitive-behavioural approach, has been found to be effective in improving interpersonal relationships and in the reduction of drinking problems (Heather *et al.* 2006).

Structured aftercare

There is evidence to suggest that planned and structured aftercare is effective in improving outcome following the initial treatment of service users with severe alcohol problems (Heather *et al.* 2006). One of the key components of psychosocial intervention is the prevention of relapse and the promoting and maintenance of abstinence. The relapse prevention programme enables the client to identify high-risk situations or triggers that can lead to problem drinking and to manage these by developing alternative coping skills and strategies (Gafoor & Rassool 1998).

Alcoholics Anonymous

Alcoholics Anonymous (AA) is a well known organisation utilised as an intervention strategy in the treatment of alcohol addiction. The only requirement for membership is a desire to stop drinking and to achieve sobriety. Members share their experiences, strengths and hopes with each other so that they can solve their common problem and help others to recover from alcohol addiction. AA created the 12-step programme, which is a set of guiding principles outlining a course of action for recovery from addiction, compulsion or other behavioural problems. The process of the 12-step programme (VandenBos 2007) includes the following:

■ Admitting that one cannot control one's addiction or compulsion.
■ Recognising a greater power that can give strength.
■ Examining past errors with the help of a sponsor (experienced member).

▪ Making amends for these errors.
▪ Learning to live a new life with a new code of behaviour.
▪ Helping others who suffer from the same addictions or compulsions.

A Cochrane Review of eight studies (Ferri *et al.* 2006), published between 1967 and 2005, measuring the effectiveness of AA, found no significant difference between the results of AA and the 12-step facilitation approaches compared to other treatments.

Harm reduction

Moderate or controlled drinking has been the health education messages for the past few decades and can be regarded as an alcohol harm reduction strategy. Alcohol harm reduction can be broadly defined as measures that aim to reduce the incidence of problem drinking and its negative consequences. Their short-term aim is to minimise the impacts of drinking alcohol and their longer term aim is to change drinking cultures – encouraging the benefits of responsible drinking and discouraging harmful drinking. The focus of harm reduction strategies is on particular risk behaviours (such as drinking and driving or binge drinking), special populations of risk groups (such as pregnant women or young people) and particular drinking contexts (such as bars and clubs). These approaches have broadened the sphere of interest in alcohol-related harm to include social nuisance and public order problems (IHRA 2003).

The recommendations of the *Sensible Drinking* report (Department of Health 1995) advise that men should not regularly drink more than 3–4 units of alcohol per day, and women should not regularly drink more than 2–3 units of alcohol per day. After heavy drinking, it is advised to have two alcohol-free days. For men over 40 and post-menopausal women, modest alcohol consumption (1 or 2 units per day) has a protective effect against coronary heart disease and strokes. This protective effect is estimated to prevent up to 22 000 deaths annually. Guidelines for sensible drinking are shown in Table 8.12.

Table 8.12 Health effects of different levels of drinking.

	Men	Women
Health benefits	1–2 units/day (>40 years old)	1–2 units/day (post-menopausal)
No significant health risks	3–4 units/day (all ages)	2–3 units/day(all ages)
Harmful effects	5 or more units/day	3 or more units/day

Summary of key points

■ Alcohol has become one of the most important risks to health.
■ Most alcohol-related deaths are caused by cirrhosis and chronic liver disease.
■ Alcohol withdrawal syndrome is a set of symptoms that individuals have when they suddenly stop drinking alcohol, following continuous and heavy consumption.
■ Both hazardous and harmful drinkers may benefit from advice, health information and brief interventions.
■ Assessment and care planning are a continuing process and a foundation for good clinical practice.
■ Screening or initial assessment is a brief process that aims to determine whether an individual has a drug and/or alcohol problem, health-related problems and risk behaviours.
■ Alcohol harm reduction aims to reduce the incidence of problem drinking and its negative consequences.

References

Anderson P. (2007) *Binge Drinking and Europe.* Institute of Alcohol Studies, London.

Anderson P. & Baumberg B. (2007) *Alcohol and Public Health in Europe.* Institute of Alcohol Studies, London.

Babor T.F. & Higgins-Biddle J.C. (2001) *Brief Intervention for Hazardous and Harmful Drinking: a manual for use in primary care.* Document No. WHO/MSD/MSB/01.6b. World Health Organization, Geneva.

Bennie C. (1998) A comparison of home detoxification and minimal intervention strategies for problem drinkers. *Alcohol and Alcoholism*, 33(2), 157–163.

Bien T.H., Miller W.R. & Tonigan J.S. (1993) Brief interventions for alcohol problems: a review. *Addiction*, 88(3), 315–336.

Castro L.A. & Baltieri D.A. (2004) The pharmacologic treatment of the alcohol dependence. *Revista Brasileira de Psiquiatria*, 26, 11. doi: 10.1590/S1516-44462004000500011 (accessed 10 June 2009).

Copello A., Orford J., Hodgson R., Tober G. & Barrett C. (2002) Social behaviour and network therapy: basic principles and early experiences. *Addictive Behaviours*, 27(3), 354–356.

Department of Health (1995) *Sensible Drinking.* Department of Health, London.

Ferri M.M.F., Amato L. & Davoli M. (2006) Alcoholics Anonymous and other 12-step programmes for alcohol dependence. *Cochrane Database of Systematic Reviews*, issue 3, article no. CD005032. doi: 10.1002/14651858.CD005032.pub2. http://www.mrw.interscience.wiley.com/cochrane/clsysrev/articles/CD005032/frame.html.

Finn D.A. & Crabbe J.C. (1997) Exploring alcohol withdrawal syndrome. *Alcohol Health and Research World*, 21(2), 149–156.

Gafoor M. & Rassool, G.H. (1998) Alcohol: community detoxification and clinical care. In G.H. Rassool (ed.) *Substance Use and Misuse: nature, context and clinical interventions.* pp. 191–199. Blackwell Science, Oxford.

Garbutt J.C., West S.L., Carey T.S., Lohr K.N. & Crews F.T. (1999) Pharmacological treatment of alcohol dependence: a review of the evidence. *Journal of the American Medical Association*, 281(14), 1318–1325.

Heather N. (1998). Using brief opportunities for change in medical settings. In W. Miller & N. Heather (eds) *Treating Addictive Behaviors*, pp. 131–148. Plenum, New York.

Heather N., Raistrick D. & Godfrey C. (2006) *A Review of the Effectiveness of Treatment for Alcohol Problems*. National Treatment Agency, London.

Hodgson C.R., Alwyn T., John B., Thom B. & Smith A. (2002) The Fast Alcohol Screening Test. *Alcohol and Alcoholism*, 37(1), 61–66.

IHRA (International Harm Reduction Association) (2003) *What is alcohol harm reduction?* www.ihra.net/alcohol (accessed 10 November 2009).

Mattick R.P. & Jarvis T. (eds) (1993) *An Outline for the Management of Alcohol Problems: quality assurance project*. Australian Government Publishing Service, Canberra.

Moore K. (2006) Alcohol and dual diagnosis. In G.H. Rassool (ed.) *Dual Diagnosis Nursing*, pp. 119–129. Blackwell Publishing, Oxford.

NICE (National Institute of Health and Clinical Excellence) (2007) *Drug Misuse: psychosocial interventions and opioid detoxification*. Clinical Guidelines No. CG51. NICE, London.

NIDA (National Institute of Drug Abuse) (2005) *Cognitive-Behavioural Therapy*. NIDA, National Institutes of Health, Bethesda, MD.

NTA (National Treatment Agency) (2006) *Review of the Effectiveness of Treatment for Alcohol Problems*. NTA Publications, London.

ONS (Office of National Statistics) (2006) *Drinking: adults' behaviour and knowledge*. Omnibus Surveys Report No. 31. HMSO, London.

ONS (Office of National Statistics) (2009) *Trend in alcohol-related deaths levelling out*. http://www.statistics.gov.uk/cci/nugget.asp?id=1091 (accessed 18 August 2009).

Rassool G.H. (2009a) *Alcohol and Drug Misuse: a handbook for student and health professionals*. Routledge, Oxford.

Rassool G.H. (2009b) Alcohol misuse: pharmacological and psychosocial interventions. In G.H. Rassool, *Alcohol and Drug Misuse. A handbook for student and health professionals*, pp. 412–424. Routledge, Oxford.

Rassool G.H. & Winnington J. (2006) Framework for multidimensional assessment. In G.H. Rassool (ed.) *Dual Diagnosis Nursing*, pp. 177–185. Blackwell Publishing, Oxford.

Royal College of Physicians (2001) *Report on Alcohol: guidelines for managing Wernicke's encephalopathy in the accident and emergency department*. Royal College of Physicians, London.

Royal College of Psychiatrists (1986) *Alcohol: our favourite drug*. Tavistock Publications, London.

Shaw, J.M., Kolesar, G.S., Sellers, E.M., Kaplan, H.L. & Sandor, P. (1981) Development of optimal treatment tactics for alcohol withdrawal. 1. Assessment and effectiveness of supportive care. *Journal of Clinical Psychopharmacology*, 1, 382–387.

Teesson M., Degenhardt L. & Hall W. (2002) *Addictions. Cinical psychology: a modular course*. Psychology Press, London.

VandenBos G.R. (2007) *APA Dictionary of Psychology*. American Psychological Association, Washington, DC.

WHO (World Health Organization) Brief Intervention Study Group (1996) A cross-national trial of brief interventions with heavy drinkers. *American Journal of Public Health*, 86(7), 948–955.

WHO (World Health Organization) (2004) *Global Status Report on Alcohol 2004*. WHO, Geneva.

WHO (World Health Organization) (2005) *Brief Intervention for Substance Use: a manual for use in primary care department of mental health and substance dependence*. WHO, Geneva.

WHO (World Health Organization) (2007) *WHO Expert Committee on Problems Related to Alcohol Consumption*. WHO Technical Report Series No. 944. WHO, Geneva.

9 Nicotine

Tobacco smoking is the single greatest cause of preventable illness and premature death and one of the most widely used psychoactive substances. It is highly addictive and the contents of cigarettes include the most toxic and carcinogenic of substances. Tobacco smoking is the second major common cause of death in the world, and is responsible for one-third of cancer cases, one-seventh of cardiovascular disease and most chronic lung disease in adults. Some of the statistics (WHO 2002) are:

■ Smoking-related diseases kill one in ten adults globally.
■ Every 8 seconds, someone dies from tobacco use.
■ Smoking is on the rise in the developing world but falling in developed nations.
■ About 15 billion cigarettes are sold daily – or 10 million every minute.
■ Among World Health Organization (WHO) regions, the western Pacific region – which covers East Asia and the Pacific – has the highest smoking rate, with nearly two-thirds of men smoking.

Addiction for Nurses By G. Hussein Rassool. © 2010 G. Hussein Rassool

The health risk factors associated with active cigarette smoking include cancer, cardiovascular disease, respiratory diseases, diabetes type 2, sexual health problems and maternal health problems. Tobacco is the single largest cause of social inequalities in health and aggravates poverty among poor smokers (Royal College of Physicians 2002). In addition to its direct health effects, tobacco leads to malnutrition, increased health care costs and premature death. It also contributes to a higher illiteracy rate, since money that could have been used for education is spent on tobacco instead (WHO 2003). Nicotine is found in chewing tobacco and the smoke from cigarettes, cigars and pipes contains thousands of chemicals, including nicotine.

The UK has high rates of death due to smoking compared to most other countries in the European Union (EU). The prevalence of regular smoking in the UK is higher among girls than in most other European countries, but UK smoking rates among boys are among the lowest in Europe (ACMD 2006). In the EU, it is estimated that tobacco consumption kills 650 000 people a year while a further 80 000 are killed by passive smoking (Europa-Eu 2007). Women under 65 in the UK have the worst death rate from lung cancer of all EU countries and the second worst death rate from heart disease, after women in Ireland. Men under 65 in the UK have a lower than average death rate from lung cancer, but the third worst death rate from heart disease, after men in Finland and Ireland (WHO 1998).

Strategy on tobacco smoking

The WHO Framework Convention on Tobacco Control (WHO FCTC) (WHO 2003) is the world's first global public health treaty and was developed in response to the globalisation of the tobacco epidemic. The treaty asserts the importance of supply and demand reduction and addresses tobacco industry marketing campaigns and cigarette smuggling, which is often coordinated by the tobacco industry in many countries. It represents a paradigm shift in developing a regulatory strategy to address addictive substances and came into force on 27 February 2005. It has since become one of the most widely embraced treaties in the United Nations' history.

In the report *Smoking Kills – a White Paper on tobacco* (Stationery Office 1999), the government's strategy is to see a reduction in smoking to improve health in Britain. The strategy in tackling tobacco smoking aims to reinforce the key goals for public health improvement and has three clear objectives:

1 To reduce smoking among children and young people.
2 To help adults – especially the most disadvantaged – to give up smoking.
3 To offer particular help to pregnant women who smoke.

A comprehensive service, provided by the National Health Service, has been implemented to help smokers to give up with added treatment, including nicotine replacement therapy.

Nicotine addiction

The WHO International Classification of Diseases 10 (ICD-10) (WHO 1992) and the Diagnostic and Statistical Manual of Mental Disorders IV (DSM-IV) (American Psychiatric Association 1995) provide a suitable framework for determining the addictive or dependent nature of nicotine and smoking. Nicotine dependence is considered to be a psychoactive substance use disorder. Applying the criteria listed in the DSM-IV or ICD-10 definitions, the features of nicotine addictions include:

▓ A strong desire to take the drug.
▓ A high priority given to drug use.
▓ Continued use despite harmful consequences.
▓ Tolerance.
▓ Withdrawal.

On present evidence, it is reasonable to conclude that nicotine delivered through tobacco smoke should be regarded as an addictive drug, and tobacco use as the means of nicotine self-administration (Royal College of Physicians 2000). Some of the characteristics of tobacco smoking are presented in Table 9.1.

Table 9.1 Characteristics of nicotine.

Street names	▓ Fags, smoke, ciggy, cancer stick, cig and many others
Legal status	▓ It is illegal to sell tobacco products to anyone under the age of 18 in the UK
Therapeutic use	▓ It has no medicinal or therapeutic uses
Sought-after effects	▓ Produces rewarding effects in the relief of stress, and in enhancing mood and performance ▓ The rapid absorption of nicotine from cigarette smoking, and the high arterial levels that reach the brain as a result, allow for rapid behavioural reinforcement from smoking
Short-term effects	▓ Headache, dizziness, insomnia, abnormal dreams, nervousness, gastrointestinal distress, dry mouth, nausea, vomiting, dyspepsia, diarrhoea and musculoskeletal symptoms ▓ Increased blood pressure ▓ Acceleration of heart rate
Long-term effects	▓ A physical dependence develops quite quickly along with psychological dependency, and quitting can be extremely difficult ▓ Smokers are more likely to suffer from heart disease, blood clots, cancer, strokes, bronchitis, circulation problems, ulcers and sexual disorders
Psychological effects	▓ Acts as a kind of mood regulator and increases pleasure ▓ Acts as a relief in highly stressful situations and periods of strong emotion ▓ Reduces aggression and irritability ▓ Increases performance and concentration on minor tasks

Harmful effects of tobacco smoke

The addictive nature of nicotine contributes to toxic or adverse effects resulting in high morbidity and mortality rates. Smoking is the most important modifiable risk factor for coronary heart disease in the young and old. The fact that smokers of whatever age, sex or ethnic group have a higher risk of heart attacks than non-smokers has been known for a quarter of a century. All these effects have also been demonstrated in those exposed to passive smoking.

The constituents of tobacco are tar, carbon dioxide and nicotine. Tar comprises 4000 different organic chemicals, including carcinogens, and on exhalation the brown sticky substance remains in the lungs, causing irritation and damage. Smokers on low tar cigarettes modify their behaviour to ensure they inhale enough smoke to achieve a satisfactory nicotine 'hit'; but by increasing their intake of nicotine, smokers also take in more tar. The average cigarette yields at least 8–20 mg of nicotine (depending on the brand), while a cigar may contain up to 40 mg of nicotine. Nicotine is broken down in the liver to produce cotinine and nicotine oxide. You can test whether or not someone has been smoking in the past day or two by screening his or her urine for cotinine. Carbon dioxide enters the bloodstream and its toxicity stems from its binding to haemoglobin to form carboxyhaemoglobin. Table 9.2 presents the harmful constituents of tobacco smoke.

Table 9.2 Harmful constituents of tobacco smoke.

Main compounds	Harms	Health problems
Tar	The various components of tar are cancer initiating and cancer accelerating	Tar in cigarette smoke paralyses the cilia in the lungs and contributes to lung diseases such as emphysema, bronchitis and lung cancer
Nicotine	This is the main toxic component of cigarette smoking and is highly addictive. It acts on the nervous system and increases the heart rate and blood pressure	Increases the stickiness of blood platelets Precipitates episodes of arrhythmia (irregular heart beat) Precipitates angina attacks
Carbon dioxide	A colourless, odourless gas, which is one of the harmful gases included in tobacco smoke Habitual smokers have a reduced amount of haemoglobin available and an increased number of red blood cells	Diseases the peripheral circulation Precipitates angina attacks

Maternal smoking during pregnancy

Maternal smoking during pregnancy exerts a direct growth-retarding effect on the fetus and delays the physical and mental development of infants. It is also associated with increased fetal and perinatal mortality and low birth weights, and has been linked to other pregnancy complications including miscarriage, stillbirth, ectopic pregnancy and cot death. The effects of smoking in pregnancy may adversely affect the child's long-term growth, behavioural characteristics and educational achievement.

Nicotine withdrawal symptoms

The withdrawal symptoms of nicotine dependence happen with a sudden stopping or reduction of smoking or other tobacco use. The physiological and psychological effects of nicotine withdrawal are presented in Table 9.3. The extent of nicotine withdrawal symptoms is dependent on the duration of smoking and number of cigarettes smoked and may begin within a few hours after the last cigarette, quickly driving people back to tobacco use.

Symptoms peak within the first few days of smoking cessation and may subside within a few weeks or may persist for months. Environmental cues such as times, places or situations associated with the pleasurable effects of smoking can make withdrawal or craving worse. Depressed smokers appear to experience more withdrawal symptoms on quitting, are less likely to be successful at quitting and are more likely to relapse.

Table 9.3 Nicotine withdrawal symptoms.

Physiological	Psychological
Dryness of the mouth	Craving
Nausea	Restlessness
Sore throat	Feeling of loneliness
Drowsiness	Inability to concentrate
Cough problems	Anger
Headache	Irritability
Tiredness	Anxiety
Postnasal drip	Depression
Bleeding in the gums	
Stomach pain	
Constipation	
Hunger pangs	
Increased appetite	
Increased weight gain	
Insomnia	
Tightness/stiffness in the chest	

Assessment and intervention strategies

The taking of a smoking history and interventions are presented in Tables 9.4 and 9.5. The expired carbon monoxide (ECO) level is measured as carbon monoxide levels are an indicator of the amount of tobacco smoke inhaled by an individual smoker (Foulds 1996). Carbon monoxide is excreted by the body quite rapidly and will reduce considerably within hours of giving up smoking. Using an ECO

Table 9.4 Taking a smoking history and interventions.

History taking	Interventions
■ Number of years as a smoker? ■ How soon after waking is the first cigarette? ■ Does the client crave a cigarette when in a no-smoking area or situation? ■ Examine any previous attempts to quit ■ Assess suitability for nicotine replacement therapy, for example no contraindications (in certain cases written permission from the client's GP may need to be obtained) ■ Ensure the client has realistic expectations of the efficacy of the treatment ■ Discuss concerns, for example withdrawal discomfort ■ Measure expired carbon monoxide levels	■ Brief interventions ■ Nicotine replacement therapy ■ Non-nicotine-based pharmacological medication

Source: adapted from Rassool, G.H. (2009) *Alcohol and Drug Misuse. A handbook for students and health professionals*, p. 428. Routledge, Oxford. Reproduced with kind permission of Taylor & Francis.

Table 9.5 Interventions and referral for smokers.

Giving up smoking	Not giving up smoking
Provide information on smoking services Give brief interventions Referral to smoking treatment services Delivery of pharmacotherapy Delivery of counselling and psychosocial support Continuing support Self-help group	Provide information on smoking services Give brief interventions

monitor where clients can see one of the positive effects of not smoking can add a major incentive towards quitting (Mills 1998).

Nurses in primary and community care should advise all patients who smoke to quit and offer a referral to a National Health Service (NHS) Stop Smoking Service. The NHS Stop Smoking Service typically combines behavioural support, delivered in a group or individual setting, with pharmacotherapy (nicotine replacement therapy or bupropion). Psychological and pharmacological interventions play an integral role in smoking cessation treatment. Self-help materials are also provided to complement the psychological interventions.

Brief interventions

The psychological techniques of brief interventions involve opportunistic advice, discussion, negotiation and encouragement interventions and typically take between 5 and 10 minutes and may include one or more of the following:

■ Simple opportunistic advice to stop.
■ Assessment of the patient's commitment to quit.
■ Pharmacotherapy and/or behavioural support.
■ Provision of self-help material and referral to the NHS Stop Smoking Services.

The National Institute for Health and Clinical Excellence (NICE 2006) has recommended that everyone who smokes should be advised to quit, and that for service users who present with a smoking-related disease the cessation advice may be linked to their medical condition. Nursing interventions for tobacco smokers are presented in Table 9.6.

Pharmacological interventions

The main forms of pharmacological treatment are nicotine replacement therapy (NRT) and the antidepressant bupropion. The aims of NRT are to reduce withdrawal symptoms by replacing the nicotine from tobacco smoking. NRT is available as:

■ Transdermal patch (varying doses, 16 hours' and 24 hours' duration).
■ Gum (2 and 4 mg).
■ Sublingual tablet (2 mg).
■ Nasal spray (0.5 mg per dose, usually administered two doses at a time).
■ Inhalator/inhaler.
■ Lozenge (1, 2 and 4 mg).

A Cochrane Review (Stead *et al.* 2008) found evidence that all forms of NRT made it more likely that a person's attempt to quit smoking would succeed. The chances

Table 9.6 Nursing interventions with smokers.

Be empathic and non-judgmental	▪ Patients may be unaware of the risks and consequences of their smoking behaviour ▪ Nurses should not condone patients admitted to hospital with a smoking-related problem ▪ Condemnation may have the counterproductive effect of both the advice and the advice giver being rejected
Be authoritative	▪ Patients recognise that true concern for their health requires that you provide authoritative advice to cut smoking or quit ▪ Be clear, objective and personal when it comes to stating the dangers of smoking
Deflect denial	▪ Some patients may deny that they smoke too much and resist any suggestion that they should cut down or quit ▪ Motivate the patient instead by giving information and expressing concern ▪ Use this information to ask the patient to explain the discrepancy between what medical authorities say and their own view of the situation. You are then in a position to suggest that things may not be as positive as they think
Engage patient in decision making	▪ It is essential that the patient participates in the process ▪ The most effective approach is to engage the patient in a joint decision-making process ▪ Ask about reasons for smoking and stress the personal benefits of quitting smoking

of stopping smoking were increased by 50–70%. Bupropion, an alternative to nicotine-based treatment, is an effective intervention and should be offered as a treatment option for patients requesting help with smoking cessation. However, bupropion is unsuitable for pregnant women and people with a history of seizures or eating disorders, for whom nicotine replacement may be considered. Bupropion is not recommended for smokers under the age of 18 years, as its safety and efficacy have not yet been evaluated for this group. Varenicline (Champix, Pfizer) has also been recommended as an option for smokers who have expressed a desire to quit smoking (NICE 2007).

Health gains and benefits of smoking cessation

▪ Improvement in overall health and health gains will be gained through smoking cessation.
▪ Nicotine withdrawal symptoms disappear after 1 month.
▪ Reduction in the risk of coronary heart disease.
▪ Reduction in the risk of stroke.

■ Reduction in risk between 30% and 50% for lung cancer has been reported after 10 years' abstinence.
■ Bladder cancer and cervical cancer risks are substantially lower after a few years of abstinence.
■ Women who stop smoking before becoming pregnant have infants of the same birth weight as those born to women who have never smoked.
■ The risk of death of former smokers compared to that of continuing smokers begins to decline shortly after giving up, until after 15 years of abstinence the risks are equalised.

Summary of key points

■ Tobacco smoking is highly addictive and the contents of cigarettes contain the toxic and carcinogenic substances.
■ The UK has high rates of death due to smoking compared to most other countries in the EU.
■ The government's strategy is to see a reduction in smoking among children and young people and to offer particular help to pregnant women who smoke.
■ Smokers could be forgiven for believing that low tar cigarettes deliver less tar to the smoker's lung.
■ The health and risk factors associated with active cigarette smoking include cancer, cardio-vascular disease, respiratory diseases, diabetes type 2, sexual health and maternal health.
■ The extent of withdrawal symptoms of nicotine is dependent on the duration of smoking and the number of cigarettes smoked.
■ The NHS Stop Smoking Service provides counselling and support to smokers wanting to quit, complementing the use of aids such as NRT and bupropion.
■ Brief intervention advice and information on treatments to aid smoking cessation should be provided.
■ The aims of NRT are to reduce the withdrawal symptoms associated with stopping smoking by replacing the nicotine from tobacco smoking.
■ Bupropion is unsuitable for some patient groups (e.g. pregnant women and people with a history of seizures or eating disorders) for whom nicotine replacement may be considered.
■ Varenicline has also been recommended as an option for smokers who have expressed a desire to quit smoking.

References

ACMD (Advisory Council on the Misuse of Drugs) (2006) *Pathways to Problems. Hazardous use of tobacco, alcohol and other drugs by young people in the UK and its implications for policy*. Home Office, London: http://drugs.homeoffice.gov.uk/publication-search/acmd/pathways-to-problems/Pathwaystoproblems.pdf.

American Psychiatric Association (1995) *Diagnostic and Statistical Manual of Mental Disorders*, 4th edn. American Psychiatric Association, Washington, DC.

Europa-Eu (2007) http://europa.eu (accessed 12 March 2009).

Foulds J. (1996) Strategies for smoking cessation. *British Medical Bulletin*, 52(1), 157–173.

Mills C. (1998) Nicotine addiction: health care interventions. In G.H. Rassool (ed.) *Substance Use and Misuse: nature, context and clinical interventions*, pp. 225–235. Blackwell Publishing, Oxford.

NICE (National Institute for Health and Clinical Excellence) (2006) *Brief Interventions and Referral for Smoking Cessation in Primary Care and Other Settings*. Public Health Guidance No. 1. NICE, London.

NICE (National Institute for Health and Clinical Excellence) (2007) *Varenicline: guidance for smoking cessation*. TA123. NICE, London.

Rassool, G.H. (2009) *Alcohol and Drug Misuse. A handbook for students and health professionals*. Routledge, Oxford.

Royal College of Physicians (2000) *A Report of the Tobacco Advisory Group*. Royal College of Physicians, London.

Royal College of Physicians (2002) *Protecting Smokers, Saving Lives*, Royal College of Physicians, London.

Stationery Office (1999) *Smoking Kills – a White Paper on tobacco*. CM4177. Stationery Office, London.

Stead L.F., Perera R., Bullen C., Mant D. & Lancaster T. (2008) Nicotine replacement therapy for smoking cessation. *Cochrane Database of Systematic Reviews*, Issue 3, article no. CD000146. doi: 10.1002/14651858.CD000146.pub3 (accessed 12 December 2008).

WHO (World Health Organization) (1992) *International Statistical Classification of Diseases and Related Health Problems*, 10th revision. WHO, Geneva.

WHO (World Health Organization) (1998) *Health for All*. Database: European region. WHO, Geneva.

WHO (World Health Organization) (2002) *Global Smoking Statistics for 2002*. WHO, Geneva.

WHO (World Health Organization) (2003) *WHO Framework Convention on Tobacco Control*. WHO, Geneva.

10 Opiates

The term 'opiate' refers to any psychoactive substance of either natural or synthetic origin that has an effect similar to morphine. Opium is the raw exudate of the opium poppy (*Papaver somniferum*) scraped from the scored seed head of the poppy, which contains a number of alkaloids including morphine and codeine. Morphine and codeine are extracted from opium, and heroin is manufactured chemically from morphine. The main sources of street heroin in the UK are the 'golden crescent' countries of Southwest Asia – mainly Afghanistan, Iran and Pakistan. Opium appears either as dark brown chunks or in powder form, and is generally eaten or smoked. The Home Office research report (Hay *et al.* 2008) estimated the prevalence of 'problem drug use', defined as use of opiates, in England to be around 273 123; this corresponds to 8.11 per thousand of the population aged 15–64 years. Changes in drug use between 2007/08 and 2008/09 showed a decrease in the use of opiates (0.2% to less than 0.05%) (Home Office 2009).

Addiction for Nurses By G. Hussein Rassool. © 2010 G. Hussein Rassool

Opiates

The characteristics of opiates are presented in Table 10.1. Other opiate analgesics appear in a variety of forms, such as capsules, tablets, syrups, elixirs, solutions and suppositories. Some of the commoner opiate drugs are codeine, heroin (diacetylmorphine), pethidine, methadone, morphine and diconal. A comparison of common opiates is presented in Table 10.2.

Heroin

Heroin is usually sold as a powder; colour ranges from white, off-white or yellowish to reddish brown, the most prevalent type now on the market. Afghansourced brown heroin is the mainstay of the UK market. It is usually dissolved in water for injection. Most street preparations of heroin are adulterated and contain only a small percentage of the drug. The adulterants include sugar, quinine or other drugs and substances. Heroin is usually sold in small quantities, typically £10 bags. In 2009, the street price of heroin was £10 for 0.15g (Druglink 2009). Habitual users of heroin generally consume from 0.5g to over 1g per day.

Multiple drug taking or poly-drug use has become a common feature with opiate users. Drugs such as benzodiazepines, amphetamines, cocaine and alcohol are frequently used in various combinations either to complement the effects of opiates or to alleviate withdrawal symptoms.

Heroin withdrawal syndrome

The initial use of heroin can result in nausea and vomiting but these unpleasant effects fade with regular use. High doses of heroin will result in drowsiness and excessive doses can produce stupor and coma and even death from respiratory failure. With regular use tolerance develops so that more heroin is needed to get the same desired effect. Physical dependence can also result from regular use.

The withdrawal syndrome from heroin may become apparent 8–24 hours after the discontinuation of sustained use of the drug. This timeframe can fluctuate with the degree of tolerance and the amount of the last consumed dose. Heroin must have been used daily for at least 2–3 weeks for physical withdrawals to occur. The withdrawal symptoms include anxiety, insomnia, diarrhoea, aches, tremor, sweating, muscular spasms, sneezing and yawning. The severity of symptoms will depend on the extent of an individual's dependence. Common symptoms of the withdrawal syndrome are presented in Table 10.3.

Drug-related overdose

Death through overdose remains a significant cause of mortality amongst heroin users in the UK, which has the highest rate in Europe (EMCDDA 2007). Heroin/ morphine used alone or in combination with other drugs accounted for the highest proportion (48%) of fatalities (Ghodse *et al.* 2006). Deaths involving methadone were more likely to be the result of illicit use (60% or more) than the use of

Table 10.1 Characteristics of opiates.

Street names	■ Brown (street heroin), China white (very pure heroin), gear, scag, scat, tiger, chi, elephant, Harry, dragon, big H, horse, junk, shit, smack, brown sugar
Legal status	■ Heroin, pethidine, morphine and methadone are class A controlled drugs. Codeine and dihydrocodeine are class B, but class A if prepared for injection. Distalgesic, dextropoxyphene and buprenorphine (Temgesic) are class C
Therapeutic use	■ The medical applications of opiates include effective relief of pain, treatment for diarrhoea and vomiting and as a cough suppressant ■ Morphine, for instance, is widely used for short-term, acute pain resulting from myocardial infarction, sickle cell crisis, surgery, fractures, burns and the later stages of terminal illnesses ■ Methadone is often prescribed to heroin addicts for maintenance or withdrawal purposes ■ Some opiates such as pethidine, morphine, dihydrocodeine and methadone are highly addictive
Non-therapeutic use	■ Heroin is swallowed, smoked, sniffed or injected either subcutaneously or intravenously ■ Smoking is often called 'chasing the dragon', or more recently 'booting' ■ Tablets are sometimes crushed and injected. If heroin powder is injected it is generally acidified using lemon juice or citric or ascorbic acid, heated with water, and then filtered prior to injecting
Sought-after effects	■ In moderate doses, opiates produce a range of generally mild physical effects apart from the analgesic effect ■ They induce euphoria, a relaxed detachment from pain and anxiety, a sense of calm, pleasure and profound wellbeing ■ They also dilate blood vessels thus giving a feeling of warmth
Adverse effects	■ Users often experience nausea or vomiting on the first occasions that they use heroin ■ Sudden withdrawal leads to anxiety, nausea, muscle pains, sweating, diarrhoea and goose flesh ■ Tolerance develops quickly so that larger amounts of the same drug are needed to produce the same effect ■ Adulterants in street heroin may increase risks of vein damage and collapse, local infections, abscesses, circulatory problems, ulcers, thrombosis, infections in heart valves and systemic infections ■ Use exposes those who share injecting equipment to blood-borne viruses including hepatitis B and C and HIV (human immunodeficiency virus) ■ Most complications arise from unsterile injections and adulterated street drugs. Heroin, taken by injection, is also a risk factor in contracting hepatitis B and C, HIV and septicaemia

Table 10.2 Features of common opiates.

Drug	Trade name	Street name	Mode of use	Duration of effect (hours)	Addictive potential
Opium		Hop, tar, big O, black stuff, Chinese molasses, Chinese tobacco, dopium, Dover's deck, God's medicine, gondola, great tobacco, joy plant, midnight oil	Smoked	4–5	High
Morphine	Generic	M, morph, painkillers, pain pills, pectoral syrup	Sniffed, injected or smoked	4–5	High
Codeine	Generic	Painkillers, pain pills	Oral	4–5	Low
Diamorphine	Heroin	Junk, smack, horse, mud, brown sugar, black tar, big H	Sniffed, injected or smoked	3–4	High
Buprenorphine	Temgesic	Tem, super Ted	Dissolved under tongue, sniffed or injected	6–8	Low
Dihydrocodeine	DF118	Duncan flockharts	Oral	4–5	Moderate
Dipipanone	Diconal	Dikes, dikies		4–5	High
Dextromoramide	Palfium			4–5	High
Methadone	Physeptone	Fizzes, dollies, juice	Oral	3–12	High
Oxycodone	Generic (Oxycontin)	Blues, oxy, painkillers, pain rills, percs, roxies, hillbilly heroin	Oral		High
Pethidine	Generic		Oral or injected	2–4	High
Dextropropoxyphene	Co-proxamol		Oral	4–5	Low

Table 10.3 Withdrawal symptoms of heroin.

▨ Sweating	▨ Diarrhoea
▨ Malaise	▨ Goose bumps
▨ Feelings of heaviness	▨ Fever
▨ Cramps	▨ Anxiety
▨ Yawning	▨ Depression
▨ Tears	▨ Insomnia
▨ Cold sweats	▨ Compulsive scratching
▨ Chills	▨ Penile erection in males
▨ Severe bone and muscle aches	▨ Extra sensitivity of genitals in
▨ Nausea and vomiting	females

prescribed drugs. A significant proportion of deaths also occurred among drug misusers who had just left prison. Deaths associated with methadone use have significantly reduced over the past 5 years, probably reflecting the implementation of supervised consumption of methadone prescriptions in the initial stages of drug treatment.

Methadone

Methadone is also known as doll, red rock, juice or script, and is commonly used as a form of treatment for opiate addiction in the UK. It is a class A drug and it is only legal for a person to possess methadone if it has been prescribed for that individual. There is a tradition in the UK of prescribing injectable methadone to opiate addicts as treatment for their addition along with injectable heroin prescribing, and this approach is known as the 'British system'. Methadone is usually prescribed as liquid syrup to be swallowed but it is also manufactured as tablets and ampoules for injection. It is easy to administer and is long acting. As with other opiates, tolerance and dependence usually develop with repeated doses. Tolerance to the different physiological effects of methadone varies. Tolerance and dependence may develop, and withdrawal symptoms, although they develop more slowly and are less acutely severe than those of morphine and heroin, are more prolonged.

Assessment of opiate dependence

There are a number of tools designed to assess the severity of opioid dependence. One of the tools is the Severity of Dependence Scale (SDS) (Gossop *et al.* 1997). This instrument is a five-item questionnaire that provides a score indicating the severity of dependence on opioids. Each of the five items is scored on a four-point

Table 10.4 Phases in the assessment of heroin dependence.

Phase 1	Phase 2	Phase 3	Phase 4
▪ How much heroin do you take a day?	▪ How many days a week do you take heroin?	▪ How much do you buy at a time?	▪ How much do you spend a week on heroin?
▪ How much did you take yesterday?	▪ How do you feel after you've taken heroin?	▪ How much do you pay per gram?	▪ How much heroin can you get by with on your worst days?
▪ How much, on average, do you take in a week?	▪ How long after you've taken some does it take before you feel rough again?	▪ How much is your habit costing you a day?	▪ How often do you score in a day?
▪ How much have you had so far today?	▪ What withdrawal symptoms are you experiencing now?	▪ How much did you take on the day you had the most last week?	▪ When was the last time you had an opiate-free day?
	▪ What do the withdrawals feel like?	▪ How many days in the last week did you have any opiates?	▪ Have there been times when you have stopped all opiate use for more than 3 days?

Source: adapted from Methadone Briefing (2009) *Section 6: assessment*: http://www.drugtext.org/library/books/methadone/section6.html. Reproduced with kind permission of Andrew Preston.

scale (0–3). The total score is obtained through the addition of the five-item ratings. The higher the score, the higher the level of dependence. The SDS takes less than a minute to complete and has been used successfully to identify degree of dependence by users of different drugs.

However, in order to assess the current level of heroin use, the assessment needs to be undertaken during several phases. A model for doing this in four phases during the course of the assessment are outlined in Table 10.4.

Intervention strategies

Detoxification

Opiate misusers must undergo a detoxification process as part of the initial stage of the treatment plan. Detoxification is the process of allowing the body to rid itself of the opiate substance while managing the symptoms of withdrawal or 'cold turkey'. It is a gradual process and can involve the use of methadone (for heroin users) for stabilisation. However, detoxification is not a treatment for heroin or opiate dependence per se. Detoxification should be a readily available treatment option for people who are opioid dependent and have expressed an informed choice to become abstinent (NICE 2007a).

The withdrawal symptoms vary with different individuals and this is influenced by the drug itself, the total intake of the drug, the duration of use and the health of the individual. Withdrawal from heroin or morphine begins 8–12 hours after the last dose of the drug and they become less over a period of 5–7 days. The detoxification process should be carried out under nursing and medical care supervision as part of a hospital or community-based programme. Methadone or buprenorphine should be offered as the first-line treatment in opioid detoxification (NICE 2007a). The most rapid regime can be carried out by incremental cuts in dose over 7–21 days although slower regimes may take several months to complete. A gradual reduction of methadone is prescribed when there are complex needs or problems. All detoxification programmes require relapse prevention strategies and psychological support after detoxification because relapse rates are high.

Psychosocial interventions

A range of psychosocial interventions are effective in the treatment of opiate dependence. Counselling and support are important both during and after withdrawal from medication. Counselling sessions can be used to explore underlying emotional conflicts and to provide an opportunity to set mutually agreed goals that will help the client to stay off drugs and improve their self-esteem. Psycho-educational interventions that give information about lifestyle changes, about reducing exposure to blood-borne viruses, and/or about reducing sexual and injection risk behaviours for people who misuse opiates should be part of the treatment package. Referral to self-help group such as Narcotics Anonymous should be facilitated for those who show an interest. Residential rehabilitation in therapeutic communities might be appropriate for those patients who are unable to achieve abstinence in other ways. For clients with coexisting substance misuse and psychiatric disorders (for example depression and anxiety), cognitive-behavioural therapy is recommended (NICE 2007b).

Case vignette

John is 35 years old and recently returned to live with his elderly parents after a period of being homeless. He has a long history of drug misuse since the age of 16 when he was taken into care by the criminal justice system for continuous petty criminal offences. He has a previous history of using multiple drugs such as crack cocaine and amphetamines on a regular basis before being introduced to heroin injecting 8 years ago. For the past year, John has been taking varying amounts of temazepam tablets, obtained through legitimate prescription and the illegal black market. He has had several admissions to the accident and emergency department with drug overdoses and other physical complications of injecting drug use. John presented to his GP complaining of panic attacks, low mood and sleeplessness.

Nursing interventions

Assessment undertaken by the multidisciplinary team indicated that John's current problems are due to benzodiazepine withdrawal and he agreed to undertake a gradual withdrawal programme from both benzodiazepines and opiates. John was provided with harm reduction information on the risks associated with injecting drugs and unsafe sexual practices. He gradually underwent detoxification from benzodiazepines and methadone. John was stabilised on 30 mg diazepam and 30 mg oral methadone linctus daily, which was gradually reduced over a 3-month period. In addition, John attended individual and group counselling sessions with support to deal with unresolved emotional difficulties. He was taught anxiety management and relaxation exercises. His self-esteem and confidence improved sufficiently enough to enable him to get a part-time job and to make changes in his lifestyle.

Summary of key points

■ The term opiate refers to any psychoactive substance, of either natural or synthetic origin, that has an effect similar to morphine.
■ There is a tradition in the UK of prescribing injectable methadone or injectable heroin to opiate addicts as treatment for their addiction and this approach is known as the 'British system'.
■ Heroin is swallowed, smoked, sniffed or injected either subcutaneously or intravenously.
■ Heroin's effects are dependent on the mode of administration.
■ In moderate doses, opiates produce a range of generally mild physical effects apart from the analgesic effect. It induces euphoria, which may wear off, but continued use avoids withdrawal symptoms.
■ Heroin dependence develops after repeated use over several weeks and sudden withdrawal leads to anxiety, nausea, muscle pains, sweating, diarrhoea and goose flesh.
■ Death through overdose remains a significant cause of mortality amongst heroin users.
■ The withdrawal syndrome from heroin may become apparent 8–24 hours after the discontinuation of a sustained use of the drug.
■ Methadone maintenance is commonly used as a form of treatment for opiate addiction in the UK because it produces similar effects to heroin or morphine.

References

Druglink (2009) *DrugScope Street Drug Trends Survey 2009*. DrugScope, London.

EMCDDA (European Monitoring Centre for Drugs and Drug Addiction) (2007) *2007 Annual Report on the State of the Drugs Problem in Europe*. EMCDDA, Lisbon: http://www.emcdda.europa.eu. (National report (2005 data) to the EMCDDA by the Reitox National Focal Point United Kingdom.)

Ghodse H., Corkery J., Oyefeso A., Schifano F., Tonia T. & Annan J. (2006) *Drug Related Deaths in the UK: annual report 2006. Drug-related deaths reported by coroners in England, Wales, Northern*

Ireland, Guernsey, Jersey and the Isle of Man and police forces in Scotland – Annual Report January–December 2005 and 17th Surveillance Report July–December 2005. International Centre for Drug Policy, St George's Hospital Medical School, London.

Gossop M., Best D., Marsden J. & Strang J. (1997) Test–retest reliability of the Severity of Dependence Scale. *Addiction*, 92(3), 353.

Home Office (2009) *Drug Misuse Declared: findings from the 2008/09 British Crime Survey, England and Wales*. Home Office Statistical Bulletin. Home Office, London.

Hay G., Gannon M., MacDougall J., Millar T., Eastwood C., Williams K. & McKeganey N. (2008) *Estimates of the prevalence of opiate use and/or crack cocaine use, 2006/07: Sweep 3 technical report*. Home Office, London. (Unpublished report.)

Methadone Briefing (2009) *Section 6: assessment*. http://www.drugtext.org/library/books/methadone/section6.html (accessed 15 June 2009).

NICE (National Institute for Health and Clinical Excellence) (2007a) *Drug Misuse: opioid detoxification*. NICE Clinical Guideline No. 52. NICE, London: www.nice.org.uk/CG52 (accessed January 2009).

NICE (National Institute for Health and Clinical Excellence) (2007b) *Drug Misuse: psychosocial interventions*. NICE Clinical Guideline No. 51. NICE, London: www.nice.org.uk/CG51 (accessed January 2009).

11 Cannabis

Cannabis is derived from a bushy plant, *Cannabis sativa*, and is used as a relaxant or mild intoxicant. Cannabis is marketed in different forms: hash or hashish (resin which is scraped from the plant and then compressed into blocks), herbal cannabis (which is a weaker preparation of dried plant material also known as marihuana) and the strongest, cannabis oil, prepared from the resin. Usually, cannabis is mixed with tobacco and smoked. Sometimes cannabis is smoked in a pipe, brewed in a drink or mixed with food.

Smoking cannabis allows the user to regulate the dose because the effect is very rapid when used in this way. Cannabis is usually retailed in packs of ounces (28 g) or fractions of ounces: 1/4 ounce (7 g) or 1/2 ounce (14 g). The retail price varies depending on whether it is sold in herbal (grass) or resin form:

- Cannabis resin: a price of £10 per eighth is still the going rate for soap-bar resin in the UK. Other varieties (e.g. Asian black, flat press) are typically £15–20 per eighth, with higher prices still for high-quality pollen and charas, and skuff when available.
- Herbal cannabis: an eighth of skunk would now cost between £20 and £25 (IDMU 2009).

Cannabis has two powerful active ingredients – THC (tetrahydrocanna-binol) and CBD (cannabidiol) – and both substances are classed as cannabinoids.

The global number of people who used cannabis at least once in 2007 is esti-mated to be between 143 and 190 million persons (UNODC 2009). The highest levels of use remain in the established markets of North America and Western Europe, although there are signs from recent studies that the levels of use are declining in developed countries, particularly among young people. In Africa and Oceania, more people presented for treatment due to problems with cannabis than any other drug (63% in Africa, 47% in Australia and New Zealand). In the UK, cannabis was the most commonly used drug in 2006/07 among all adults and young adults, and in 2008/09, with 7.9% of adults having used it in the last year (Information Centre 2008).

The characteristics of cannabis are presented in Table 11.1.

Cannabis as a gateway drug

The theory that cannabis use can lead to the use of hard drugs is not supported by evidence that the use of one drug actually causes people to use another (escala-tion theory). Generally, people who smoke cannabis are more likely to use other drugs, and people who smoke tobacco and drink are more likely to try cannabis. Tobacco smoking is a better predictor of the use of hard drug use than smoking cannabis (Ellgren 2007). The RAND study (Morral *et al.* 2002) demonstrated that associations between cannabis and hard drug use could be expected even if can-nabis use has no gateway effect. Instead, the associations can result from known differences in the ages at which youths have opportunities to use cannabis and hard drugs, and known variations in the willingness of individuals to try any drugs.

Cannabis withdrawal syndrome

There is now a growing consensus of the existence of a cannabis-dependence syndrome that is consistent with other classic psychoactive drugs of addiction. There are stronger risks of developing tolerance and experiencing withdrawal symptoms with cannabis cessation due to the increasing potency of the drug. Symptoms of cannabis withdrawal first appear in chronic users within the first 8 hours and are the most noticeable during the first 10 days, but withdrawal symp-toms may last as long as 45 days. The withdrawal from cannabis is identifiable by behavioural and emotional distress. Withdrawal symptoms from cannabis can be characterised as the opposite to the intoxicating effects of the drug. For example, instead of hunger, a loss of appetite, and instead of drowsiness, an inability to sleep. Some additional symptoms of cannabis withdrawal can include headache, nausea, anxiety, paranoia, irritability or aggression; the symptoms are usually

Table 11.1 Characteristics of cannabis.

Street names	■ Dope, draw, blow, resin, grass, skunk
Legal status	■ Cannabis is controlled under the Misuse of Drugs Act as a class C drug
	■ It is illegal to cultivate, produce, supply or possess the drug, unless a Home Office licence has been issued for research use or other special purposes
	■ It is an offence to allow any premises to be used for cultivating, producing, supplying, storage or smoking of cannabis
Therapeutic use	■ Cannabis is indicated for the treatment of anorexia associated with weight loss in patients with AIDS (acquired immune deficiency syndrome), and to treat mild to moderate nausea and vomiting associated with cancer chemotherapy
Short-term use	■ The effects derived depend to a large extent on the expectations, motivation and mood of the user
	■ The effects of cannabis usually start just a few minutes after smoking and last from about 1 hour to several hours depending on how much is consumed
	■ Some users experience an intense feeling of relaxation
	■ The following are common effects: talkativeness, bouts of hilarity, relaxation and greater sensitivity to sound and colour
	■ There is no hangover of the type associated with alcohol use
	■ Whilst under the influence of cannabis, concentration and mental and manual dexterity are impaired, making tasks such as driving or any procedure requiring accuracy or precision both difficult and dangerous
Long-term use	■ Like tobacco, frequently and chronically inhaled cannabis smoke probably causes bronchitis and other respiratory problems and may also contribute to the development of lung cancer
	■ Generally people who smoke cannabis are more likely to use other drugs, and people who smoke tobacco and drink are also more likely to try cannabis
	■ However, there is no evidence that the use of one drug actually causes people to use another (escalation theory)
	■ While there is little evidence that cannabis can produce a physical dependence, regular use can produce a psychological need for the drug and some individuals may come to rely on it as a 'social lubricant'
	■ Perceptual distortion may also occur, especially with heavy use
	■ If the drug is used while an individual is anxious or depressed, these feelings may be accentuated leading to a feeling of panic
	■ People chronically intoxicated on cannabis appear apathetic, sluggish and neglectful of their appearance
	■ There may be particular risks for people with respiratory or heart disorders
	■ Heavy use, particularly if strong varieties such as some forms of skunk are used regularly, can lead to psychosis
	■ Heavy users of cannabis with personality disturbance or psychiatric problems may precipitate a temporary exacerbation of symptoms

Table 11.2 Withdrawal symptoms from cannabis.

Common withdrawal symptoms	Uncommon withdrawal symptoms
Anxiety	Tremors
Irritability	Nausea
Restlessness	Vomiting
Physical tension	Occasional diarrhoea
Decrease in appetite	Excessive salivation
Perspiration	
Increased aggression/anger	
Sleep disturbances	
Moodiness	
Anorexia	

strongly experienced. During this period the cravings to use cannabis are strongest. Common and uncommon withdrawal symptoms are presented in Table 11.2.

Assessment

Assessment may comprise taking a drug history of the current presentation of an individual's cannabis pattern of use. The assessment should focus on the current pattern of cannabis use, the quantities and associated problems. In order to ascertain the level of dependency, it is important to ask about experiences of withdrawal symptoms or any psychological complications. An outline of the assessment procedure is shown in Table 11.3. A mental state assessment should be undertaken when psychiatric symptoms are evident.

There are a number of self-administered instruments in the assessment of cannabis use. Cannabis-dependent individuals presenting for treatment typically report cannabis craving. The Marijuana Craving Questionnaire (MCQ) (Heishman *et al.* 2003) consists of four factors that characterise cannabis craving: compulsivity, emotionality, expectancy and purposefulness. The MCQ (the 47-item or 12-item versions) can be used to measure cue-elicited craving in cannabis-dependent individuals presenting for treatment. For the diagnosis of cannabis dependence, the Diagnostic and Statistical Manual of Mental Disorders IV (DSM-IV) criteria should be used. The severity of dependence scale (Gossop *et al.* 1997) has also been adapted to assess the psychological aspects of cannabis dependence.

There is a World Health Organization (WHO) standardised and validated screening instrument: ASSIST, Alcohol, Smoking and Substance Involvement Screening Test (Henry-Edwards *et al.* 2003), which is used to identify persons with hazardous or harmful use of a range of psychoactive substances including tobacco, alcohol, cannabis, cocaine, amphetamine-type stimulants, sedatives, hallucinogens, inhalants, opioids and 'other drugs'. ASSIST is short and easy to use and can be administered quickly in primary care settings. It has been validated in many countries with differing cultures, languages and health systems.

Table 11.3 Assessment of cannabis use.

▦ **Statement of the need/problem**	Consider the individual's concerns, issues, needs or problems
▦ **Current cannabis use**	Type, quantity and frequency
▦ **Pattern of drug or alcohol use**	Details of drug taking for the past week/month
▦ **Current use of other substances**	Prescribed, illicit or over-the-counter drugs
▦ **Level of dependence**	Any withdrawal symptoms Evidence of increasing tolerance
▦ **Associated problems**	Any psychological or legal problems
▦ **Risk behaviours**	Sexual behaviour when intoxicated
▦ **Periods of abstinence/relapse**	Duration and periods of abstinence (voluntary or enforced) Reasons for lapse or relapse
▦ **Sources of help**	Social support systems Statutory agencies Local authorities Voluntary agencies Self-help groups
▦ **Coping strategies and strengths**	Previous strategies in coping with use of the drug Achievements, strengths and positive aspects of the individual

Source: Rassool G.H. & Winnington J. (2006) Framework for multidimensional assessment. In G.H. Rassool (ed.) *Dual Diagnosis Nursing*, p. 181. Blackwell Publishing, Oxford.

ASSIST consists of eight questions and provides information about:

■ The substances people have ever used in their lifetime.
■ The substances they have used in the past 3 months.
■ Problems related to substance use.
■ Risk of current or future harm.
■ Dependence.
■ Injecting drug use.

Intervention strategies

There are number of strategies that can be used in the management and care of cannabis dependence. However, there is a widespread consensus that cannabis dependence does not require treatment because the withdrawal syndrome of cannabis is so mild that most users can quit or cease to use without requiring medical assistance. There are a number of cannabis users who seek help and treatment for

their addiction. The treatment strategies include brief interventions, health education, harm reduction, assistance with withdrawal symptoms, relapse prevention
and psychological interventions.

Brief interventions

Research into effective brief interventions for substance use have found that the
features of FRAMES (feedback, responsibility, advice, menu of options, empathy
and self-efficacy (confidence for change)) appear to contribute to their effectiveness (Bien *et al.* 1993; Miller & Sanchez 1993).

The provision of personally relevant feedback is a key component of brief interventions. Feedback can include information about the individual's cannabis use,
information about personal risks associated with current drug use patterns, and
general information about cannabis-related risks and harms. There may also be a
link between the current presenting symptoms and cannabis use. It is important
to inform the patient about the link as part of feedback and to emphasise their
responsibility for their own behaviour. The key component of effective brief interventions is the provision of clear advice regarding the harms associated with
continued use of cannabis. The users should also be provided with self-help
resources to enable them to cut down or stop their cannabis use. The final component of effective brief interventions is to encourage patients' confidence that
they are able to make changes in their substance use behaviour.

Motivational interviewing

Rollnick and Miller (1995) defined motivational interviewing as 'directive, client-
centred counselling for eliciting behaviour change by helping clients to explore
and resolve ambivalence'. They described it as more focused and goal-directed
than non-directive counselling, and said the counsellor should take a directive
approach to the examination and resolution of ambivalence, which is its central
purpose.

Motivational interviewing is employed when patient show no or little commitment to change their behaviour. Motivational interviewing is based on the premise
that the main obstacle to changing drug or alcohol use and associated behaviour
patterns is a lack of motivation; it follows that if motivation to change can be
enhanced then behaviour change will be more likely (Baker & Reicher 1998). It is
a technique that does not require an in-depth counselling knowledge, and involves
a non-judgmental approach, open-ended questioning and reflective listening. It is
used in such a way as to raise the patient's self-esteem, self-efficacy and increase
awareness of their problems. The four principles of motivational interviewing are:
(i) express empathy; (ii) develop discrepancy; (iii) roll with resistance; and
(iv) support self-efficacy. Various tools and strategies have been developed to help
apply these principles and these include pencil and paper exercises, structured

Table 11.4 Components of a relapse prevention programme.

Components	Interventions
Identification of high-risk situations and triggers for cravings	Role play
How to say no to buying or using cannabis	Self-talk, distracting activities, diary of periods of craving
Development of skills to cope with cravings	Development of a personal emergency plan to identify steps for dealing with relapses
Identifying alternative pleasurable activities	Problem-solving skills, relaxation training, identification and modification of negative thoughts
Learning to cope with lapses	
Develop management of low mood and anger	
Creation of a personal self-help sheet	Documenting the benefits of not using cannabis, risks of using it and high-risk situations

Source: Marlatt G.A. & Gordon J.R. (1985) *Relapse Prevention: a self-control strategy for the maintenance of behaviour change.* Guilford Press, New York.

questions and focused reflections (Mason 2006). McCambridge and Strang (2004) reported reductions in the use of cannabis, cigarettes and alcohol among young people in the UK after just one session of motivational interviewing.

Relapse prevention

Relapse prevention is a cognitive-behavioural technique centred on the teaching of coping skills. There is good evidence of the effectiveness of specific relapse prevention in the treatment of drug and alcohol problems and psychosocial functioning (NTA 2006a, 2006b). The techniques used to teach coping skills include identification of specific situations where coping inadequacies occur, and the use of instruction, modeling, role play and behavioural rehearsal. Exposure to stressful situations is gradually increased as adaptive mastery occurs. An important part of any plan should include assertiveness work and social inclusion. The components of a relapse prevention programme are shown in Table 11.4.

Assistance with withdrawal symptoms

Most users of cannabis do not require medication assistance during detoxification or withdrawal from cannabis. However, a minority of patients may need help with pharmacotherapy to alleviate the mild symptoms of cannabis withdrawal. Some patients may experience severe agitation, restlessness, irritability, insomnia or nightmares and may be prescribed benzodiazepine 4 mg tds for a short duration. This should be complemented with psychosocial and educational interventions. There are no pharmacological therapies for cannabis misuse and there has been limited research in this area.

Case vignette

J.D. is a 25-year-old unemployed man who was referred to a local alcohol and drug service by his general practitioner. He reported smoking ten joints of skunk cannabis each day, usually alone. In addition, he drinks alcohol on a recreational basis. J.D. presented as a pleasant and cooperative young man. He was casually dressed and neat in appearance. There was no evidence of intoxication or withdrawal. He was relaxed throughout the interview and his speech was spontaneous and coherent. However, he described feeling low in mood, irritable and unable to have regular sleep at night. His urinalysis was confirmed positive for cannabis. His goal was to stop smoking cannabis completely. He was offered a number of psychological intervention sessions by the community psychiatric nurse.

Psychological and nursing interventions

J.D. was offered six sessions of motivational interviewing. Through the process of engagement the nurse developed and maintained a therapeutic alliance with J.D. A non-judgmental and empathic approach was adopted to help J.D to identify his own reasons for stopping his cannabis use. Attempts to have a confrontational and judgmental approach may exacerbate the potential for clients to disengage with treatment services. Issues about stopping the use of cannabis or the harm caused by cannabis use were not addressed directly until the end of the engagement process when a working alliance has developed. Guidelines that help promote engagement (Rethink & Turning Point 2004) with the patient are presented in Table 11.5.

J.D. had insight into his use of cannabis and recognised that he smoked cannabis in an attempt to relax and 'chill out'. He reported having a lack of motivation at times and suffered from mild social anxiety. The social anxiety made him reluctant to go out and socialise with his peer groups. As a result of this amotivational factor, he has not been able to complete his engineering course and would like to achieve this goal. J.D. stated that he was contemplating change but was unable to do so due to low self-efficacy and self-confidence. Assessment all too often focuses only on the individual's negative aspects of substance misuse such as an individual's weakness, risks and problems. The inclusion of an assessment of positive aspects of the individual regarding substance misuse may highlight and enhance the self-efficacy and self-esteem of the individual. The position of strengths should focus on strategies that the individual has 'successfully' used in previous attempts to manage substance misuse. In this context, the nurse supported J.D.'s self-efficacy by highlighting a past strength: in the past, J.D. had succeeded in giving up cigarettes. If he could stop smoking cigarettes, he could also stop smoking cannabis. This positive approach may enable the individual to engage with services with less resistance and also influence the individual's coping strategies and treatment outcomes (Rassool & Winnington 2006).

The nurse taught J.D. a number of coping strategies such as delaying the first joint of the day for as long as possible and the use of other recreational activities to displace the cannabis use. Physical exercise such as jogging and swimming were used as distractors. The nurse also taught J.D. about restructuring his negative thoughts into positive ones. During the maintenance phase of J.D.'s new behaviour, a number of high-risk situations for cannabis use were identified, and activities and thoughts that could help him to cope with any cravings at these times were explored. After subsequent support and counselling, J.D. managed to stop smoking cannabis. He reported feeling less social anxiety, more optimistic about his future, and more confident that he could continue to abstain from cannabis use.

Table 11.5 Promoting engagement.

■ Motivate clients to see the benefits of the treatment process – this requires a clear idea of what they need and value
■ Have a non-confrontational, empathic and committed approach
■ Offer help with meeting initial needs such as food, shelter, housing and clothing
■ Provide assistance with benefit entitlements
■ Provide assistance with legal matters
■ Involve family or carers wherever possible
■ Meet clients in settings where they feel safe; this may be more constructive than expecting them to come to services

Source: Rethink & Turning Point (2004) *Dual Diagnosis Toolkit: mental health and substance misuse*. Rethink and Turning Point, London.

Summary of key points

■ Cannabis is the most commonly used psychoactive substance in the world.
■ In England and Wales, cannabis remains the most widely used drug.
■ Herbal cannabis, also known as marihuana or grass, is a weaker preparation of dried plant material.
■ Cannabis has two powerful active ingredients: THC and CBD (cannabidiol) and both substances are classed as cannabinoids.
■ It is an offence to allow any premises to be used for cultivating, producing, supplying, storage or smoking of cannabis.
■ The alleged relationship between cannabis and more illicit drugs, as proposed by the gateway theory, is methodologically flawed.
■ The effectiveness of a therapeutic alliance is crucial to the delivery of any treatment intervention and patient outcomes.
■ Brief interventions comprise of a single brief advice or several short (15–30 minutes) brief counselling sessions.
■ Motivational interviewing is 'directive, client-centred counselling for eliciting behaviour change by helping clients to explore and resolve ambivalence'.
■ Patients may need support to identify risks associated with their substance misuse and a relapse prevention plan is based on the identified risk factors.

References

Baker A. & Reichler R. (1998) *Motivational Interviewing. Clinical Skills Series: effective approaches to alcohol and other drug problems*. Visual Education, Suffolk, UK.

Bien T.H., Miller W.R. & Tonigan S. (1993) Brief intervention for alcohol problems: a review. *Addiction*, 88(3), 315–336.

Ellgren M. (2007) *Neurobiological effects of early life cannabis exposure in relation to gateway hypothesis*. Karolinska Institute, Karolinska: http://diss.kib.ki.se/2007/978-91-7357-064-0 (accessed 15 March 2009).

Gossop M., Best D., Marsden J. & Strang J. (1997) Test–retest reliability of the Severity of Dependence Scale. *Addiction*, 92(3), 353.

Heishman S.J., Evans R.J., Singleton E.G., Levin K.H., Copersino M.L. & Gorelick D.A. (2003) Reliability and validity of a short form of the Marijuana Craving Questionnaire. *Drug and Alcohol Dependence*, 102(1–3), 35–40.

Henry-Edwards S., Humeniuk R., Ali R., Monteiro M. & Poznyak V. (2003) *Brief Intervention for Substance Use: a manual for use in primary care*. (Draft version 1.1 for field testing.) World Health Organization, Geneva: http://www.idmu.co.uk/cannabis-prices/cannabis-price-trends-94-08.html.

IDMU (Independent Drug Monitoring Unit) (2009) *Cannabis prices, 2008*. http://www.idmu.co.uk/prices.htm (accessed 18 April 2010).

Information Centre (2008) *Statistics on drug misuse: England*. http://www.ic.nhs.uk/webfiles/publications/Drugmisuse08/Statistics%20on%20Drug%20Misuse%202008%20final%20format%20v12.pdf.

Marlatt G.A. & Gordon J.R. (1985) *Relapse Prevention: a self-control strategy for the maintenance of behaviour change*. Guilford Press, New York.

Mason P. (2006) Motivational interviewing. In G.H. Rassool (ed.) *Dual Diagnosis Nursing*, pp. 253–260. Blackwell Publishing, Oxford.

McCambridge J. & Strang J. (2004) The efficacy of single-session motivational interviewing in reducing drug consumption and perceptions of drug-related risk and harm among young people: results from a multi-site cluster randomized trial. *Addiction*, 99(1), 39–52.

Miller W. & Sanchez V. (1993) Motivating young adults for treatment and lifestyle change. In G. Howard (ed.) *Issues in Alcohol Use and Misuse by Young Adults*, pp. 55–81. University of Notre Dame Press, Notre Dame, IN.

Morral A.R., McCaffrey D.F. & Paddock S.M. (2002) Reassessing the marijuana gateway effect. *Addiction*, 97(1), 1493–1504.

NTA (National Treatment Agency) (2006a) *Treating Drug Misuse Problems: evidence of effectiveness*. NTA Publications, London.

NTA (National Treatment Agency) (2006b) *Review of the Effectiveness of Treatment for Alcohol Problems*. NTA Publications, London.

Rassool G.H. & Winnington J. (2006) Framework for multidimensional assessment. In G.H. Rassool (ed.) *Dual Diagnosis Nursing*, pp. 117–185. Blackwell Publishing, Oxford.

Rethink & Turning Point (2004) *Dual Diagnosis Toolkit: mental health and substance misuse*. Rethink and Turning Point, London.

Rollnick S. & Miller W.R. (1995) What is motivational interviewing? *Behavioural and Cognitive Psychotherapy*, 23(4), 325–334.

UNODC (United Nations Office of Drugs and Crime) (2009) *World Drug Report 2009*. UNODC, Vienna: www.unodc.org.

12 Psychostimulants

Amphetamines and cocaine are stimulants available in a variety of tablets and capsules, sometimes in combination with other drugs. Khat is also a psychostimulant and is an evergreen shrub. Psychostimulants are psychoactive substances that cause an increase in activity in various parts of the central nervous system, producing restlessness, arousal and stimulating behaviour, and are often referred to as 'uppers'. Psychostimulants can be legal or illegal psychoactive substances. Legal stimulants include caffeine, a mild stimulant which is considered relatively safe, and nicotine (found in tobacco products). Historically, stimulants were used to treat asthma and other respiratory problems, obesity, neurological disorders and symptoms of depression. Stimulant drugs included in this chapter are: amphetamines, cocaine, khat, ecstasy and amyl nitrite. Around one in five adults (19.2%) in the UK have at some point taken stimulant drugs, and nearly one in 20 had taken these drugs in the last year (4.4%) (Home Office 2009).

Amphetamines

Amphetamine, dextroamphetamine and methamphetamine are collectively referred to as amphetamines. During the past decades, amphetamine became popular as a recreational drug and performance enhancer amongst young people. Recently amphetamine has experienced a revival in its uses. The most common type is amphetamine sulphate, which is relatively easy to produce. Amphetamines can cause feelings of euphoria, enhanced self-confidence and self-awareness, greater energy and heightened alertness.

Most 'street stimulants' are illicitly manufactured amphetamine sulphate powder. Illicit amphetamine heavily diluted with adulterants (often to 15% purity) is easily available and is often manufactured in home-made laboratories in a matter of hours, with the main ingredient being pseudo-ephedrine (a cold remedy) mixed in a cocktail of about 15 chemicals. This process is highly toxic and dangerous. Crystal amphetamine (methamphetamine hydrochloride), the street form of the drug methamphetamine, comes in clear, chunky crystals and is heated and smoked. Smokeable methamphetamine is usually called ice and is an off-white, grey or pinkish powder which is usually smoked in a glass pipe. In 2007, amphetamine was being sold at £9.80 per gram in the UK (Druglink 2007). Amphetamine base is more expensive, typically £20–30 per gram. The 2008/09 British Crime Survey report (Home Office 2009) indicates that 1.2% of 16–59 year olds reported using amphetamines in England and Wales. Their characteristics are presented in Table 12.1. In most amphetamines users, the effects of the drug disappear when they stop using the drug.

Routes of administration

The intensity of amphetamines is based on the amount of drug taken and the routes of administration. Amphetamines can be swallowed, sniffed, smoked or injected (by crushing the tablets). In very low doses, amphetamines increase attention spans and decreases impulsiveness, whereas in higher doses, it decreases appetite and results in weight loss. In its oral form, the user experiences increased wakefulness and physical activity, and decreased appetite. If smoked and injected, the user immediately experiences an intense 'rush' (also called a 'flash') that causes intense pleasure but only lasts a few minutes. With repeated use, stimulants can decrease dopamine levels, dampening users' ability to feel pleasure and the

Table 12.1 Characteristics of amphetamines.

Street names	▨ Speed, whizz, sulph, uppers, ice, crystal, glass, amph, billy, sulphate
Legal status	▨ All amphetamines and similar stimulants are prescription-only drugs under the Medicines Act ▨ Most are also controlled under the Misuse of Drugs Act with the exception of some mild stimulants ▨ Amphetamine, dexamphetamine, methylamphetamine, phenmetrazine and methylphenidate are in class B, but if prepared for injection the increased penalties of class A apply ▨ Diethylpropion and other amphetamine-like stimulants are class C
Therapeutic use	▨ It is commonly used to treat attention-deficit hyperactivity disorder (ADHD) in adults and children ▨ It is also used to treat symptoms of traumatic brain injury, symptoms of narcolepsy and chronic fatigue syndrome ▨ Amphetamines can also be used as supplement to antidepressant therapy in depressive conditions
Sought-after effects	▨ Amphetamines create arousal and the user feels more energetic, confident and cheerful ▨ Heart and respiratory rate are speeded up, pupils widen and appetite lessens ▨ The experience of these effects creates the possibility of psychological dependence ▨ As the individual's energy is depleted the predominant feelings may be anxiety, irritability and restlessness ▨ Snorting produces effects within 3–5 minutes, and oral ingestion takes 15–30 minutes to produce the effects ▨ These methods produce a euphoric effect, but only the rapid-onset methods produce an intense rush
Short-term effects	▨ Short-term physiological effects vary greatly, depending on the dosage used and the method in which the drug is taken ▨ The effects of a single dose last about 3–4 hours, leaving the user feeling tired and depleted. It can take a couple of days for the body to fully recover
Long-term effects	▨ Amphetamine may cause violent behaviour, anxiety, confusion and insomnia ▨ Heavy users may also display a number of psychotic features, including paranoia, auditory hallucinations, mood disturbances and delusions known as amphetamine psychosis ▨ Paranoid delusions may result in homicidal or suicidal thoughts ▨ Heavy prolonged use also exposes the individual to the risk of cardiovascular problems ▨ Amphetamines can also cause a variety of problems, including rapid heart rate, irregular heartbeat, stroke, high blood pressure, shortness of breath, nausea, vomiting, diarrhoea and physical collapse ▨ There may also be an increase in body temperature and convulsions, which can be lethal if not treated as an emergency

Table 12.2 Withdrawal symptoms of amphetamines.

▩ Cravings	▩ Hyperventilation
▩ Nausea	▩ Convulsions
▩ Irritability	▩ Irregular heart beat
▩ Depression	▩ Insomnia
▩ Loss of energy	▩ Depression
▩ Sweats	▩ Long periods of
▩ Fatigue	sleep
▩ Decreased libido	▩ Paranoia
▩ Decreased self-confidence	▩ Delusions

development of tolerance. Chronic users of amphetamines typically snort or resort to drug injection to experience the full intensity of the drug's effects with the added risks of infection, vein damage and higher risk of overdose.

Amphetamine withdrawal syndrome

The use of amphetamines is highly addictive, and, with chronic abuse, tolerance develops very quickly. Many amphetamine users will repeat the amphetamine cycle by taking more of the drug during withdrawal. There is evidence for the existence of an amphetamine dependence syndrome, arrayed along a continuum of severity (Topp *et al.* 1995). Withdrawal, although not physiologically threatening, is an unpleasant experience. How severe and prolonged these withdrawal symptoms are depends on the degree of abuse. The key withdrawal symptoms of amphetamines are presented in Table 12.2.

Cocaine

Cocaine, a white powder derived from the leaves of the Andean coca shrub, is a psychoactive drug with powerfully stimulant properties. In Europe and North America, the most common form of cocaine is a white crystalline powder. There are three forms of cocaine: cocaine hydrochloride, freebase and crack cocaine. Freebasing consists of smoking cocaine base (or crack). Crack cocaine (rocks, ready wash, ice, base, freebase, stones) is whitish in colour and looks like irregular lumps of sugar. Crack is made by heating cocaine hydrochloride with baking soda or ammonia in water. Alcohol is often mixed with cocaine to produce coca-ethylene, which is highly toxic.

In recent years, there has been considerable concern regarding rises in cocaine use in recreational settings (e.g. discos and clubs) and among young people in general in some European countries. Cocaine is the second most commonly used illicit drug in Europe, after cannabis (EMCDDA 2007). Worldwide, the total number of people who used cocaine at least once in 2007 is estimated to range between 16 and 21 million (UNODC 2009). The largest market remains North America, followed by Western and Central Europe and South America. Some African countries, notably in western and southern Africa, appear to show rising levels of cocaine use, although data are sparse (UNODC 2009). In England and Wales, cocaine powder was the next most commonly used drug (after cannabis) – 3.0% of 16–59 year olds reporting use of it in 2008/09 (Home Office 2009).

Cocaine powder is generally used by socially integrated recreational users, while crack cocaine remains very rare, being mainly consumed by more marginalised groups (e.g. the homeless or sex workers). In many cases, cocaine users are poly-drug users, often consuming cocaine with alcohol and tobacco, with other illicit drugs such as other stimulants and cannabis, or with heroin (EMCDDA 2007). Cocaine is a stimulant but is not normally prescribed therapeutically for its stimulant properties, although it is used as a local anaesthetic. The street name, legal aspects, therapeutic effects and sought-after effects are presented in Table 12.3.

The physical and psychological effects of cocaine based on low to moderate use, excessive use and chronic use are presented in Table 12.4.

Routes of administration

The intensity and the duration of the effects of cocaine are influenced by the route of administration. A traditional way of taking cocaine is chewing coca leaves mixed with an alkaline substance (such as lime or bicarbonate). The effects of chewing coca leaves is felt within 15–20 minutes; with the increase in alertness, awareness and feeling of wellbeing there is an increase in activity or the desire to do something. The effect of chewing is strong at the start but it disappears progressively and it is necessary to increase the intake slowly to maintain the effect. Alternatively, coca leaves can be infused in liquid and consumed like tea. With oral administration, cocaine takes approximately 30 minutes to enter the bloodstream. Given the uptake of cocaine in the bloodstream and the slow rate of absorption, the effects are reached approximately 60 minutes after cocaine is administered and these effects are prolonged for approximately 60 minutes after their peak is attained. Snorting, sniffing or blowing (insufflation) is the most common method of ingestion of cocaine. Snorting cocaine produces maximum physiological effects within 40 minutes and an activation period of between 5 and 10 minutes, which is similar to oral use of cocaine. With smoking freebase, the cocaine is absorbed immediately into the blood, reaching the brain in about 5 seconds. The peak of the freebase rush is rapid and the high typically lasts 5–10 minutes. These effects are similar to those that can be achieved by injecting cocaine hydrochloride but without the risks associated with injecting drug use.

Injecting cocaine is very risky; people who inject drugs put their lives in danger more than other drug users. Injecting cocaine can end up being a frequent activity and because pain is deadened around the injecting site, veins become damaged

Table 12.3 Characteristics of cocaine.

Street names	■ Coke, Charlie, C, white, Percy, snow, toot
Legal status	■ Cocaine, its derivative salts and the leaves of the coca plant come under class A of the Misuse of Drugs Act ■ A doctor must be licensed by the Home Office before prescribing cocaine
Therapeutic use	■ Freud expected that cocaine would be used as a substitution therapy for morphine addiction and as a euphoriant in cases of melancholia ■ Cocaine has previously been used as a local anaesthetic in ophthalmology and dentistry ■ Cocaine was also used in the treatment of asthma, cramps, mountain sickness, sea sickness, vomiting in pregnancy and vomiting
Sought-after effects	■ A rapid feeling of intense high ■ Increased alertness and energy ■ A feeling of wellbeing ■ Delayed hunger and fatigue ■ Increased confidence ■ Stimulated sex drive
Adverse effects	■ Several quickly repeated doses can lead to extreme agitation, panic attacks and feelings of restlessness, irritability and anxiety ■ Chronic use of cocaine results in ongoing rhinitis (runny noses) and damage to the nasal septum ■ Many users report a burning sensation in the nostrils after cocaine's anaesthetic effects wear off ■ Cocaine has an effect on the constriction of blood vessels and prevents adequate blood supply to that area ■ Cocaine users may also experience paranoia, auditory hallucination or a full-blown cocaine psychosis ■ The long-term use of cocaine can cause debilitation due to lack of sleep and food, leading to lowered resistance to illness generally

very quickly (trafford.knowcocaine.co.uk.). It is always safer to sniff cocaine than injecting it.

■ Sharing, lending or borrowing injecting equipment can spread hepatitis B, hepatitis C and HIV (human immunodeficiency virus).
■ Poor injecting technique or dirty equipment can damage veins and cause infection and blood poisoning.
■ Lowered tolerance and the unknown purity of street drugs can result in an overdose.

A highly dangerous practice is the injection of a mixture of heroin and soluble cocaine (known as snowballing or speedballing). Coca ethylene is produced when

Table 12.4 Physical and psychological effects of cocaine.

Dose	Physical effects	Psychological effects
Low to moderate doses	Loss of appetite Dry mouth Tachycardia Raised heart rate Hypertension Sweating Dilated pupils Reduced appetite Reduced need for sleep Impaired motor skills Reduced lung function Erratic or violent behaviour Increased desire for sex	Euphoria Sense of wellbeing Impaired reaction time Increased self-confidence Suspiciousness Increased sensory awareness Sense of superiority
Excessive doses	Convulsions Heart failure Stroke Cerebral haemorrhage Respiratory arrest Exhaustion	Anxiety Irritability Insomnia Depression Paranoia Aggressiveness Delusions Disorientation Indifference Reduced psychomotor function
Chronic use	Destruction of nasal septum (snorting) Nasal eczema (snorting) Chest pains Muscle spasm Respiratory problems (smoking) Contraction of infection (injected cocaine) Abscesses (injected cocaine) Weight loss Malnutrition Sexual impotence	Tolerance Psychological dependence Cocaine psychosis

alcohol and cocaine are consumed together. Coca ethylene is active in the brain, and has a similar effect to cocaine, but the subjective perception of the cocaine 'high' and its heart effects are not increased – instead they decline in intensity.

Cocaine withdrawal syndrome

Cocaine users can develop a tolerance to the euphoric effects of cocaine, which makes it necessary to take more and more cocaine to get the same desired effect.

Table 12.5 Signs and symptoms of crack cocaine withdrawal.

■ Depression
■ Insomnia
■ Anorexia
■ Fatigue
■ Irritability
■ Restlessness
■ Psychiatric disorders
■ Craving

Cocaine causes both physical and psychological dependence, the severity of which depends on the route of drug administration. Psychological dependence is more of a problem than physical withdrawal symptoms. It is more severe when the drug has been injected or smoked. Withdrawal leads to strong cravings and drug-seeking behaviour, followed by a withdrawal syndrome. The signs and symptoms of crack cocaine withdrawal are presented in Table 12.5.

Stages in cocaine withdrawal

Cocaine withdrawal generally occurs in three phases: the 'crash', 'withdrawal' and 'extinction' (Table 12.6). Not all cocaine users go through the three distinct phases as this may be influenced by the level of cocaine consumption, the set and the setting.

During cocaine withdrawal there is no physical evidence as with heroin withdrawal. Crack cocaine withdrawal is not as physically evident nor are there visible physical symptoms like the vomiting and shaking that accompanies heroin withdrawal or the seizures and delusions that can follow alcohol withdrawal.

Khat

Khat acts as a social lubricant in the Yemen, Ethiopia and Somalia. It is an evergreen shrub (*Catha edulis*), a 2–4 m flowering evergreen shrub that grows in parts of East Africa and the Middle East. Chewing khat predates the use of coffee and is used in a similar social context. It is transported to the UK by air and is generally preferred fresh as the leaves from the plant are most powerful when recently picked. The prevalence data on the use of khat range from 34% to 67% of the Somali community in the UK who identify themselves as current users of khat (ACMD 2005). Khat users appear to have very low levels of use of other drugs or alcohol. There is no evidence that khat use is a gateway to the taking of other stimulant drugs, although there is high associated tobacco use (ACMD 2005).

The main active substances in khat are cathine and cathinone and these are closely related to amphetamine but are of less potency. As the leaves mature or

Table 12.6 Stages in cocaine withdrawal.

Crash	▪ Occurs in the first few days after a sudden stop in cocaine use ▪ Even first-time users of cocaine can experience the crash, depending on dosage and length of use ▪ The withdrawal symptoms experienced can last between 9 hours and 4 days ▪ Agitation ▪ Depression ▪ Anxiety ▪ Anorexia ▪ Intense craving for cocaine ▪ Uncontrollable appetite ▪ Insomnia or prolonged, but disturbed, sleep ▪ Extreme fatigue and exhaustion
Withdrawal	▪ The withdrawal phase may last up to 10 weeks from the end of the crash ▪ In the middle phase of withdrawal, severe cravings for cocaine are experienced ▪ Craving may be reinforced by cues such as cocaine paraphernalia or other environmental cues ▪ Physiological responses such as runny nose, taste sensations and fidgetiness may occur ▪ Other withdrawal symptoms during this phase include: low energy anhedonia (inability to feel pleasure) anxiety angry outbursts
Extinction	▪ For some cocaine users, extinction lasts for at least 6 months and for others it is indefinite ▪ Some cocaine users may experience craving when faced with strong cues (people, places or objects) ▪ Relapse is high because of continued cravings

dry, cathinone is converted to cathine, which significantly reduces its stimulatory properties. Cathinone is approximately ten more times more potent than cathine and is only present in fresh leaves. The street names, legal aspects, sought-after effects and adverse effects are presented in Table 12.7.

Khat is used for its stimulant effects. The effects are similar to, but less intense than, those of methamphetamine or cocaine. Fresh leaves are chewed and dried leaves are smoked, made into a paste and chewed, or brewed in tea. Users usually chew about 50 g (2 ounces) of leaves or stems for a number of hours, swallowing the juice. Dryness of the mouth is caused by the juice so large amounts of liquid are also drunk. Effects start about 30 minutes into chewing and finish up to 2 hours after stopping.

Table 12.7 Characteristics of khat.

Street names	■ Quat, qat, kat, qat, chat, gat, graba, tohai, tschat, mirraa
Legal status	■ The khat plant is legal, but its active ingredients cathinone and cathine are class C
Sought-after effects	■ Khat generally produces talkativeness, mild euphoria and hallucinations. In many countries it has social and cultural significance and is mostly used as a social stimulant on festive occasions
Adverse effects	■ Periods of lethargy, irritability and general hangover ■ Dependence can develop and heavy use can be problematic ■ Nausea, vomiting, mouth ulcers, abdominal pain, headache, palpitations, increased aggression and hallucinations can occur ■ Continued use can lead to cycles of sleeplessness and irritability and can in the longer term lead to psychiatric problems such as paranoia and possibly psychosis ■ Digestive problems such as constipation and stomach ulcers have been reported frequently to affect regular users

Effects

Effects start after approximately 30 minutes, with stimulation and talkativeness. This is followed by a relaxed and introspective state that can last up to 5 hours, often with insomnia. This is then followed by periods of lethargy, irritability and general hangover. Dependence can develop and heavy use can be problematic. Nausea, vomiting, mouth ulcers, abdominal pain, headache, palpitations, increased aggression and hallucinations can occur. Continued use can lead to cycles of sleeplessness and irritability and can in the longer term lead to psychiatric problems such as paranoia and possibly psychosis. Digestive problems such as constipation and stomach ulcers have been reported frequently to affect regular users. Khat is also often used with tobacco and hypnosedatives such as benzodiazepines, which brings additional associated risks. The physical and psychological risks associated with khat are presented in Table 12.8.

Ecstasy

Ecstasy or 3,4-methylenedioxymethamphetamine (MDMA), is a synthetic, psychoactive drug with hallucinogenic and amphetamine-like properties. It is often categorised as a hallucinogen, as in some respects it resembles LSD (lysergic acid diethylamide). The main use of ecstasy has been as a 'dance' or 'rave culture' drug. Ecstasy usually comes in tablet form, powder or in capsules with different shapes

Table 12.8 Risks of khat use to physical and psychological health.

Risks to physical health	Risks to psychological health
Increase in blood pressure	Low mood
Risk factor for oral cancer	Dependence
Risk factor for myocardial infarction	? Psychosis
Affects reproductive heath	
Delivery of low birth weight babies	
Lower sperm motility	
Increased libido	
Decreased libido (chronic use)	
Risks from residual pesticides	

and colours. The strength and contents of ecstasy tablets cannot be known accurately as all ecstasy available on the street is produced in unregulated black market laboratories. Ecstasy is sometimes cut with amphetamines, caffeine and other substances. Ecstasy tablets are also crushed and snorted or taken in a liquid form through injection, but swallowing is the most common method of use.

A UK 2007 survey (DrugScope 2007) reported that the bottom had fallen out of the ecstasy pill market with the average street price of a pill now as low as £2.40, with pills most commonly sold in batches of three to five for £10. The use of ecstasy by adults aged between 16 to 59 years old in 2008 was estimated at 1.8% (Home Office 2009). Ecstasy users may test positive for amphetamines in the standard drug test. The street names, legal aspects, therapeutic uses, sought-after effects and adverse effects are presented in Table 12.9.

Effects

The effects of ecstasy usually begin within 20 minutes of taking the drug, and may last up to 6 hours. The physiological effects that can develop include dilated pupils, a tingling feeling, tightening of the jaw muscles, raised body temperature, increased heart rate, muscle tension, involuntary teeth clenching, nausea, blurred vision, rapid eye movement, faintness and chills or sweating. The psychological effects can include anxiety, panic attacks, depression, sleep problems, drug craving, confused episodes and paranoid or psychotic states. The physiological and psychological effects of ecstasy are presented in Table 12.10.

Tolerance and dependence

Ecstasy is not physically addictive in the way that drugs like cocaine, nicotine and heroin are. Many users, however, may develop tolerance to the effects of ecstasy.

Table 12.9 Characteristics of ecstasy.

Street names	■ E, Adam, XTC, doves, 'Dennis the Menace', 'Rhubarb and Custard', New Yorkers, love doves, disco burgers, pills, brownies, Mitsubishi's, Rolex's, dolphins, phase 4
Legal status	■ Ecstasy is a class A drug
Therapeutic use	■ Ecstasy has been used as an appetite suppressant ■ It has been used as an adjunct to various types of psychotherapy in order to facilitate the therapeutic process ■ Used to some extent with terminally ill patients in order to help them come to terms with their situation and to ventilate their feelings more easily
Sought-after effects	■ Effects start about 20–60 minutes after use and can last several hours ■ Users describe ecstasy as making them empathic, producing a temporary state of openness with an enhanced perception of colour and sound ■ The user experiences euphoric feelings, and feelings of empathy, relaxation and meaningfulness ■ Tactile sensations are enhanced for some users, making physical contact with others more pleasurable
Effects (three phases)	■ There is the 'coming up' effect when the user experiences a sudden amphetamine-like rush ■ This rush is accompanied by mild nausea. It is immediately followed by a plateau of intoxication where the user may feel good, happy and relaxed ■ The final phase is the 'coming down' where the user may feel physically exhausted, depressed or irritable
Adverse effects	■ Adverse effects of ecstasy include tiredness, confusion, anxiety and depression ■ With higher doses the user can feel anxious and confused, and coordination can be impaired, making driving or similar activities very dangerous ■ If taken regularly over a period of a few days the user can experience panic attacks, temporary paranoia or insomnia ■ The use of this drug may be more hazardous for individuals with heart conditions, hypertension, blood clotting disorders, a history of seizures or any type of psychiatric disorder

Table 12.10 Immediate and adverse effects of ecstasy.

	Physiological effects	Psychological effects
Immediate effects	Increase in physical energy Increased heart rate Increased body temperature Increased blood pressure Nausea Sweating Ataxia Involuntary jaw clenching Teeth grinding Loss of appetite Dilated pupils	Relaxation Euphoria Empathy Increase in emotional energy Increased ability to interact with others Increase in confidence Heightened sensitivity Increased responsiveness to touch Changes in perception Feelings of insight Anxiety Short-term memory lapses
Adverse effects	Decreased ability to perform tasks Tachycardia Hyperthermia Hyponatraemia Nystagmus Convulsions Vomiting Motor rituals Headaches	Increased restlessness Confusion Depression Sleep problems Attentional dysfunction Panic attacks Floating sensations Impairment of cognitive functions Poor memory recall Increased anxiety Depressed mood Depersonalisation Irrational or bizarre behaviour Hallucinations. Catatonic stupor

Frequent ecstasy use increases tolerance very quickly. Increasingly higher doses are needed to reach an 'acceptable' high. The use of larger amounts will increase the severity of undesirable effects, rather than increase the pleasurable effects. To avoid the build-up of tolerance, long breaks should be left between uses (at least 2 months).

Amyl and butyl nitrite

Amyl and butyl nitrites are stimulant and are known collectively as alkyl nitrites. To users, alkyl nitrites are known as poppers. Amyl and butyl nitrites are clear, yellow, volatile and inflammable liquids with a sweet smell when fresh and are chemically related to nitrous oxide or laughing gas. When stale, the drug

Table 12.11 Characteristics of amyl and butyl nitrite.

Street names	▦ Poppers
Legal status	▦ Butyl nitrite is not classified as a drug and has no restrictions on its availability under current medicine or drug legislation ▦ However, other laws such as the Offences Against the Persons Act 1861 may be used to restrict distribution of these substances
Therapeutic use	▦ Medically, amyl nitrite has been used in the treatment of angina and as an antidote to cyanide poisoning ▦ Butyl nitrite has no therapeutic medical uses
Sought-after effects	▦ Once inhaled, the effects are virtually instantaneous and last for 2–5 minutes. The blood vessels dilate, heart rate increases and blood rushes to the brain ▦ Those using the drug to enhance sexual pleasure report a slow sense of time, prolonged sensation of orgasm and the prevention of premature ejaculation ▦ Alkyl nitrites are also used for relaxation of the anal sphincter, easing anal intercourse
Adverse effects	▦ The are a number of effects of using nitrites, including: dizziness, relaxation of muscles, increased heart rate, low blood pressure, feeling flushed, blurred vision, headaches, vomiting, burning feeling (mouth and nose) and death due to existing heart problems or low blood pressure ▦ Anyone with cardiovascular problems, glaucoma and anaemia should avoid using nitrites ▦ There appear to be no serious long-term effects of the drug as it is excreted rapidly from the body in healthy individuals but there are reports that it may suppress the immune system ▦ Use after alcohol, cannabis or cocaine may worsen the adverse effects

degenerates to a smell often described as 'smelly socks'. The vapour is inhaled through the nose or mouth from a small bottle or tube. In the UK, drugs such as butyl nitrite are on sale in sex shops, pubs, bars and clubs. As a street drug, butyl nitrite comes in small bottles with screw or plug tops. In 2008, the use of amyl nitrite by 16–59 year old in England and Wales was estimated to be 1.4% (Home Office 2009). The characteristics of poppers are presented in Table 12.11.

Tolerance to amyl nitrite

Tolerance to the drug develops within 2–3 weeks of regular use, but after a few days of abstinence this tolerance is lost. There are no reports of withdrawal

Table 12.12 Immediate and long-term effects of amyl nitrite.

Immediate effects	Long-term effects
Dizziness	Reduced resistance to infections
Relaxation of muscles	Suppressed immune system
Increased heart rate	
Low blood pressure	
Feeling flushed	
Blurred vision	
Headaches	
Vomiting	
Burning feeling (mouth and nose)	
Death (due to existing heart problems or low blood pressure)	

symptoms or psychological dependence. The immediate and long-term effects of nitrites are presented in Table 12.12.

Mephedrone

Mephedrone, also known as 4-methylmethcathinone (4-MMC), is a synthetic stimulant drug and research chemical of the phenethylamine, amphetamine and cathinone chemical classes. It emerged on the so-called 'legal highs' market and reportedly produces stimulant effects that are comparable to those of similar drugs such as MDMA (ecstasy). Mephedrone, nicknamed meph, has been sold in high street 'head shops' (which sell bongs and rolling paraphernalia) and on the Internet as a plant food or 'research chemical'. A typical price in the UK is £15 per gram. Effects include euphoria, alertness, talkativeness and feelings of empathy. However, users can have the same adverse effects of stimulants and become anxious or paranoid.

The drug is currently controlled under the Misuse of Drugs Act and banned in the UK as a class B substance. Anyone found in possession of mephedrone could face 5 years in prison. Dealing the drug will carry a maximum sentence of 14 years.

Assessment of psychostimulants

Assessment and management of a patient presenting with acute psychostimulant toxicity can be a demanding and potentially dangerous activity. For those psychostimulant users who are unwilling to accept that they have a problem, a non-confrontational and emphatic approach is more likely to nudge the users into engagement with the services. Obtaining a good history of drug use, including where, how and why the stimulant has been used is very important. The assessment should include a through physical examination and state mental examination. This is supported by urinalysis to confirm the use of stimulants.

Signs of recent psychostimulant drug usage may include:

- Agitation and pacing, with rapid speech and repetitive movements.
- Tachycardia.
- Sweaty palms and flushed/diaphoretic skin.
- Clenched jaw or muscle rigidity.
- Hypervigilance and paranoia.
- Dilated (mydriatic) pupils reacting sluggishly to light.
- Long-term users may display signs of poor nutrition, have sores on their face, arms or legs, or have needle marks or thrombophlebitis.
- Patients may become acutely hyperthermic with temperatures above 39.5°C.

Intervention strategies

Nursing interventions

Patients on stimulants may crash into a critical condition without warning. Even first-time users of cocaine can experience a crash, depending on dosage and length of use. Stimulant users may become extremely agitated and violent, displaying erratic and unpredictable behaviour. Patients may also experience panic attacks, delirium, irritability, confusion and tactile, auditory and visual hallucinations. When addressing an agitated or paranoid patient, it is important to talk in a calm, even, clear voice and avoid prolonged eye contact. Make sure that instructions given are short and unambiguous. When interacting with a potentially volatile patient it may be helpful to avoid reacting to the situation. The effective approach is to respond to the needs of the patient.

Physical restraints may be necessary to ensure both safety to the staff and the patient, and to control the situation so that physical assessment and interventions can be undertaken. However, physical restraints should not be used until other interventions have failed and the patient is at imminent or perceived risk to themselves or others. Clear protocols should be should be established in dealing with potentially aggressive or abusive patients, and staff should be trained in this competence. Set firm boundaries with respect to aggressive or counterproductive behaviour.

Try to give positive information on what you will do to help the patient. Management of toxic reactions is presented in Table 12.13. However, the management will depend on the patient's condition on presentation. The medical and

Table 12.13 Management of toxic reactions of stimulants.

Priority	Nursing intervention
Respiration	Maintain airway, breathing and circulation
Control elevated body temperature	Hydration, cold water, ice
Discomfort	Aim to decrease discomfort
Control seizures	Administration of prescribed intravenous
Induce sleep or reduce anxiety and	diazepam
agitation	Administration of prescribed diazepam
Managing psychotic symptoms	Administration of prescribed antipsychotics
Psychological support	Reassurance, support and comfort
Control of environment	Minimal stimulation
Managing psychosocial problems	Counselling
Plan for lapse and relapse	Relapse prevention; use and dangers of
Prepare for harm reduction strategies	using stimulants
	Safer injecting practices; safer sexual
	behaviours

psychological problems associated in the toxicity of psychostimulants drugs and their interventions are presented in Table 12.14.

Psychosocial interventions

Psychosocial interventions have most commonly been used to treat psychostimulants users, in part because of the absence of a strong evidence base demonstrating the effectiveness of pharmacotherapies. Kamieniecki *et al.* (1998) examined the use of in-patient programmes, therapeutic communities, 12-step programmes, peer interventions, behavioural strategies, cognitive-behavioural interventions and acupuncture with psychostimulant users. They reported that those non-pharmacological interventions that demonstrated the most efficacy were relapse prevention, cue exposure/response prevention, and multifaceted behavioural treatment. However, it was noted that many of the interventions had not been properly evaluated.

Baker and colleagues (2005) recommended that a stepped care approach should be adopted. This involves the provision of intervention tailored to individual needs, with the employment of more intensive interventions as indicated by the degree of dependence and severity of problems experienced by the individual. Thus, those presenting at non-treatment settings may be involved in a structured assessment of amphetamine use and related problems, provided with self-help materials, and their use and harms regularly monitored. Those presenting to treatment settings may be offered two or more sessions of cognitive-behavioural therapy, depending on the extent of use and coexisting problems (e.g. depression).

Table 12.14 Medical and psychological management.

Problem	Interventions
Serotonin syndrome (ecstasy)	■ May develop in patients using psychostimulants, particularly MDMA ■ Life-threatening symptoms such as extreme hyperthermia, muscle rigidity, hyper- or hypotension, seizures and coma ■ Patient may develop hyperkalaemia, acidosis, rhabdomyalysis or renal failure ■ Hyperthermia above 39.5°C will require rapid cooling ■ Intravenous volume resuscitation to correct dehydration and hypotension ■ Strict fluid balance, aiming for urine output of 1.5–2 ml/kg/h
Cardiovascular (amphetamines)	■ Ischaemic chest pain due to myocardial vasoconstriction ■ Treatment is as per chest pain protocol (including oxygen and sublingual nitroglycerine to relieve vasoconstriction) ■ *Except* aspirin should be avoided if the patient has prolonged hypertension due to increased risk of intercerebral haemorrhage and beta-blockers should be avoided as they may exacerbate adverse effects ■ Benzodiazepines should be considered to manage anxiety and prolonged hypertension
Cerebrovascular (cocaine and amphetamines)	■ Increases the risk of stroke and cerebral haemorrhage ■ Management includes ABC (airway, breathing, circulation), supportive care and early head CT (computerised tomography) scan if deterioration in neurological status ■ Seizures should be treated with benzodiazepines. Aspirin should be avoided as above
Hyponatraemia (ecstasy)	■ May occur as a result of excessive fluid intake (MDMA) ■ Patient may become confused and have seizures ■ May be treated with fluid restriction or in severe cases with i.v. hypertonic saline ■ Careful monitoring of fluid balance and electrolytes is essential
Psychosocial problems	■ Complex medical and psychosocial problems ■ Referral to specialist drug and alcohol services

Source: adapted from Department of Health and Ageing (1998) *Models of Intervention and Care for Psychostimulant Users*. Monograph No. 32. Department of Health and Ageing, London.

Case vignette

Julie, a 26-year-old female, was taken to A&E by a friend in the early hours of the morning. She presented with persistent headache, lethargy and unexplained weight loss. In addition, she was preoccupied by concerns of an individual being after her who wished her harm. She works as a lawyer and has been a regular cocaine user and had been taking cocaine intranasally. She has an active work and social life, and consequently tends to eat poorly. Julie was assessed and it was recommended that Julie be admitted to the acute psychiatric unit for observation with a referral to the Community Drug and Alcohol Team. After a short stay on the ward, she gradually gained insight into the cause of her persecutory beliefs and benefits from the opportunity to talk through her experiences with her key worker.

Activity 12.1

- How would you engage Julie to undertake specialist treatment?
- How would you manage the acute psychosis?
- What symptomatic drug treatment does Julie need during the withdrawal period?
- What psychological intervention would be suitable in order to focus her attention on her cocaine use?
- How would you enable Julie to deal with lapse and relapse?

Summary of key points

- Amphetamine, dextroamphetamine and methamphetamine are collectively referred to as amphetamines.
- Chronic users of amphetamines typically snort or resort to drug injection to experience the full intensity of the effects of the drug.
- Injecting cocaine has the added risks of infection, vein damage and a higher risk of overdose.
- Smoking cocaine base is a more potent way of administration than snorting and produces a 'rush' similar to the experience of injecting cocaine.
- Many cocaine and crack users also take other drugs, including heroin. Alcohol is often mixed with cocaine to produce coca-ethylene, which is highly toxic.
- Withdrawal leads to strong craving and drug-seeking behaviour followed by a withdrawal syndrome.
- Cocaine withdrawal generally occurs in three phases: the 'crash', 'withdrawal' and 'extinction'.
- Khat generally produces talkativeness, mild euphoria and hallucinations.
- Nausea, vomiting, mouth ulcers, abdominal pain, headache, palpitations, increased aggression and hallucinations can occur with khat use.
- The user of ecstasy experiences euphoric feelings and feelings of empathy, relaxation and meaningfulness.
- The adverse effects of ecstasy include tiredness, confusion, anxiety and depression.
- Some people may develop tolerance to the effects of ecstasy; using larger amounts will increase the severity of undesirable effects, rather than increase the pleasurable effects.

References

ACMD (Advisory Council on the Misuse of Drugs) (2005) *Khat (Qat): assessment of risk to the individual and communities in the UK*. Home Office, London.

Baker A., Lee N.K., Claire M. *et al*. (2005) Brief cognitive behavioural interventions for regular amphetamine users: a step in the right direction. *Addiction*, 100(3), 367–378.

Department of Health and Ageing (1998) *Models of Intervention and Care for Psychostimulant Users*. Monograph No. 32. Department of Health and Ageing, London: http://www.health.gov.au/internet/main/publishing.nsf/Content/phd-drugs-mono32-cnt.htm.

Druglink (2007) *Average UK National Street Drug Price*. Druglink, London: http://www.drugscope.org.uk.

DrugScope (2007) *Street Drug Trends Survey 2007*. Drugscope, London: www.drugscope.org.uk.

EMCDDA (European Monitoring Centre for Drugs and Drug Addiction) (2007) *Cocaine and crack cocaine: a growing public health issue*. EMCDDA Statistical Bulletin: http://stats06.emcdda.europa.eu/en/homeen.html (accessed 21 June 2009).

Home Office (2009) *Drug Misuse Declared: findings from the 2008/09 British Crime Survey, England and Wales*. Home Office Statistical Bulletin. Home Office, London: http://www.homeoffice.gov.uk/rds/pdfs09/hosb1209.pdf.

Kamieniecki G., Vincent N., Allsop S. & Lintzeris N. (1998) *Models of Intervention and Care for Psychostimulant Users*. Monograph Series No. 32. National Centre for Education and Training on Addiction, Commonwealth Department of Health and Family Services, Canberra.

Topp L., Mattick R.P. & Lovibond P.F. (1995) *The nature of the Amphetamine Dependence Syndrome: appetitive or aversive motivation?* NDARC Technical Report No. 30. National Drug and Alcohol Research Centre, University of New South Wales, Sydney.

UNODC (United Nations Office of Drugs and Crime) (2009) *World Drug Report 2009*. UNODC, Vienna: www.unodc.org.

13 Other Psychoactive Substances

This chapter deals with a group of substances known as hallucinogens or hallucinogenic drugs, hypnosedatives, over-the-counter drugs and smart and eco drugs. The term hallucinogens refers to a diverse group of drugs, natural or synthetic, that induce an alteration in perception, thought, emotion and consciousness. Lysergic acid diethylamide, known as LSD, is derived from a synthetic alkaloid (ergot). Other hallucinogens include psilocybin (liberty cap mushrooms), *Amanita muscaria* (fly agaric mushrooms), morning glory seeds, mescaline (peyote cactus), PCP (phencyclidine) and ketamine. In England and Wales, the use of hallucinogens (LSD and magic mushrooms) in 2008 was estimated at 0.6%, as was the use of ketamine (Home Office 2009).

Addiction for Nurses By G. Hussein Rassool. © 2010 G. Hussein Rassool

LSD (lysergic acid diethylamide)

LSD is an odorless, colorless and tasteless powder derived from a fungus that grows on rye and other grains. LSD usually comes in the form of liquid, tablets or capsules, squares of gelatine or blotting paper. The blotter paper is divided into small decorated squares, with each square representing one dose. LSD can be swallowed, sniffed, injected or smoked. LSD is taken by mouth in extremely small doses (50–150 µg), usually on small paper squares. The effects tend to start about half an hour after taking it and last up to 12 hours or sometimes even longer, depending on the dosage. The legal status, therapeutic use, sought-after effects and adverse effects are presented in Table 13.1. Table 13.2 lists the physical and psychological effects of LSD.

Tolerance, dependence and withdrawal

Tolerance to the euphoric and psychedelic effects of hallucinogens develops after three or four daily doses. Any tolerance developed quickly goes away once regular use is stopped. Frequent, repeated doses of LSD are unusual and therefore tolerance is not commonly seen. There is no physical dependence or withdrawal symptoms associated with recreational use of LSD; it is not considered an addictive drug since it does not produce compulsive drug-seeking behaviour.

GHB (gammahydroxybutyrate)

GHB is a colourless liquid, with a slightly salty taste, and is a central nervous depressant. It is produced as a result of fermentation and so is found in small quantities in some beers and wines, particularly fruit wines, with limited effect. The drug is usually sold in small 30 ml plastic containers (costing approximately £15) and consumed in capfuls. It is sometimes sold as 'liquid ecstasy' although it is not related to ecstasy. The drug can take anything from 10 minutes to an hour to take effect and the effects can last from 1.5 to 3 hours or even longer. Users of GHB enjoy an alcohol-like or ketamine intoxication with potent positive sexual effects. GHB can lead to respiratory depression and death, especially when combined with alcohol. Its characteristics are presented in Table 13.3.

As the dosage increases there are adverse effects that can lead to disorientation, nausea, confusion, a numbing of the muscles or muscle spasms and vomiting. At high doses, convulsions, coma and respiratory collapse can occur. The drug also lowers blood pressure and in some cases people find breathing difficult. Combining GHB and any other sedative, especially alcohol, is extremely dangerous. When in a GHB-induced sleep, convulsions can occur, often requiring emergency care. Driving or operating machinery while under the influence of GHB increases the risk of physical injury or accident to the user and to others. The long-term effects

Table 13.1 Characteristics of LSD.

Street names	■ Acid, microdots, dots, tabs, trips
Legal status	■ LSD is a class A controlled drug
Therapeutic use	■ Hallucinogens have been investigated as potential therapeutic agents in treating several disorders including depression, obsessive-compulsive disorder, alcohol dependence and opiates addiction ■ In recent times, LSD has been used occasionally in psychotherapy
Sought-after effects	■ The effects of the drug are dependent on the user's prior experience, mood, expectations and setting ■ A moderate dose will produce profound alterations in mood, sensation and consciousness, intensified sensory experiences and perceptual distortions ■ Confusion of time, space, body image and boundaries can occur with what have been called the blending of sight and sound ■ The user may 'see' sounds and 'hear' colours ■ Mushrooms are similar to LSD, but the trip is often milder and shorter
Adverse effects	■ Panic, confusion, impulsive behaviour, unpleasant illusions (bad trip), flashbacks and possible precipitation of psychotic reactions ■ In a 'bad trip', the user may experience strong feelings of anxiety, paranoia, panic or fear ■ Hallucinations can be unpleasant, such as the feeling of insects crawling on the skin ■ A lack of control and ability to stop the experience can cause panic ■ LSD can produce physiological effects including elevated heart rate, increased blood pressure, dilated pupils, higher body temperature, sweating, loss of appetite, sleeplessness, dry mouth and tremors ■ If taken in a large enough dose, the drug produces delusions and visual hallucinations ■ Feelings of panic, paranoia and fear can lead to risky behaviour that can cause injury, such as running across a busy street or jumping out of a window ■ There is a strong risk of precipitating a relapse in those already susceptible to schizophrenia

of GHB remain unknown. The drug has been referred to in the media as a date rape drug, in much the same way as alcohol and Rohypnol.

Dependence and withdrawal

Regular use of GHB can cause physical dependence. The withdrawal symptoms will subside after 2–21 days depending on the doses and frequency of use.

Table 13.2 Physical and psychological effects of LSD.

	Physical effects	Psychological effects
Short-term effects	Dilated pupils Lowered body temperature Nausea Vomiting Profuse sweating Rapid heart rate Hypertension Convulsions Loss of appetite Sleeplessness Impaired coordination Risk of accidents	Heightened senses (sight, sound and touch) Distorted perception of depth, time and the size and shape of objects Hallucinations (stationary objects appear to be moving) Anxiety Depression Dizziness Disorientation Paranoia Panic
Long-term effects	? Organic brain damage	Tolerance Flashbacks Disorientation Anxiety Distress Prolonged depression Increased delusions Psychosis

Withdrawal from GHB may cause symptoms similar to acute withdrawal from alcohol or barbiturates (delirium tremens) and can cause convulsions, paranoia and hallucinations. Withdrawal effects may include:

■ Insomnia.
■ Restlessness.
■ Anxiety.
■ Tremors.
■ Sweating.
■ Loss of appetite.
■ Tachycardia.
■ Chest pain.
■ High blood pressure.
■ Muscle and bone aches.
■ Sensitivity to external stimuli
■ Inability to sleep.

Ketamine

Ketamine, in powder form, appears similar to that of pharmaceutical cocaine and can act as a depressant and a hallucinogenic. It is sold in either powdered or liquid

Table 13.3 Characteristics of GHB.

Street names	▓ Liquid ecstasy, GBL, BDO, GBH, blue nitro, midnight blue, renew trient, reviarent, somatopro, serenity, enliven
Legal status	▓ GHB is categorised as a class C drug in the UK, with dealers facing up to 5 years in prison and possession punishable by up to 2 years
Therapeutic use	▓ GHB has been used historically as a general anaesthetic, as a hypnotic in the treatment of insomnia, to treat depression and to improve athletic performance ▓ In Italy, GHB is used in the treatment of acute alcohol withdrawal and medium- to long-term detoxification
Sought-after effects	▓ Effects range from relaxation to sleep at low doses ▓ A small capful can make you feel uninhibited, exhilarated, relaxed and feeling good with the effects lasting as long as day, although it is difficult to give a clear 'safe' dose, as the concentration of the liquid varies ▓ Regular alcohol users break down GHB faster than people who do not drink alcohol
Effects: recreational dose	▓ Euphoria ▓ Increased enjoyment of movement and music ▓ Increased libido ▓ Increased sociability ▓ Intoxication
Effects: higher dose	▓ Nausea and vomiting ▓ Desire to sleep ▓ Giddiness ▓ Slurred speech ▓ Dizziness ▓ Respiratory depression ▓ Drowsiness ▓ Agitation ▓ Visual disturbances ▓ Depressed breathing ▓ Amnesia ▓ Convulsions ▓ Unconsciousness ▓ Death

form. Ketamine can be inhaled, injected or mixed in drinks. The effects are evident in about 10–15 minutes and last about 1 hour. It is also possible to smoke ketamine mixed with cannabis and tobacco. The drug is often mixed with other psychoactive substances such as cocaine and ecstasy to enhance their potency. With intravenous use, the onset of the effects of ketamine is immediate and reaches peak effect within minutes. The street names, therapeutic effects, sought-after effects and adverse effects are presented in Table 13.4.

An investigation by DrugScope (2009) has revealed concerning trends in the use of the class C drug ketamine, with users taking higher doses of the drug and more people injecting the substance. Some drug services are also reporting an increase in the number of young people using ketamine. The British Crime Survey (Home Office 2008) reported that the use of ketamine amongst 16–59 year olds in England and Wales was 0.40% in the year 2007/08; that is, approximately 113000 adults used ketamine during this period. Ketamine is odourless and tasteless, so it can

Table 13.4 Characteristics of ketamine.

Street names	■ Special K, green, super K, vitamin K
Legal status	■ Ketamine is a class C drug, which means that it is illegal to possess it and to supply it
Therapeutic use	■ It is currently used in human anaesthesia and veterinary medicine
Sought-after effects	■ Ketamine users report sensations ranging from a pleasant feeling of floating to being separated from their bodies ■ A giddy euphoria occurs with lower doses, often followed by bursts of anxiety or mood lability ■ Some ketamine users' experiences involve a terrifying feeling of almost complete sensory detachment that is likened to a near-death experience ■ These experiences, similar to a 'bad trip' on LSD, are called K-holes
Adverse effects	■ Higher doses produce a withdrawn state (disassociation); when doses are higher still, disassociation can become severe (known as a K-hole) with ataxia, dysarthria, muscular hypertonicity and myoclonic jerks ■ With very high doses, coma and severe hypertension may occur; deaths are unusual. Acute effects generally fade after 30 minutes ■ Ketamine may impair memory and aggravate existing psychosis, anxiety or depression. Prolonged use may cause disorientation and gradual detachment from the world ■ Ketamine produces only mild respiratory depression and cardiovascular status is usually unaffected ■ In addition, ketamine has both analgesic and amnesic properties and is associated with less confusion, irrationality and violent behaviour than PCP

Table 13.5 Physiological and psychological effects of ketamine.

Dose level	Physiological effects	Psychological effects
Low	Vertigo Ataxia Slurred speech Slow reaction time	Euphoria
Higher	Analgesia Movement difficult Muscular hypertonicity Hypertension Mild respiratory depression Coma	Amnesia Dissociation (K-hole) Disorganised thinking Speech unintelligible Altered body image Feeling of unreality Visual hallucinations

be added to beverages without being detected, and it induces amnesia. A summary of the physiological and psychological effects of ketamine are shown in Table 13.5.

Psilocybin

Psilocybin ('magic mushrooms') is usually sold as dried mushrooms or in substances made from mushrooms. In its pure form, psilocybin is a white powder. The most common type of mushroom is the liberty cap. They can be eaten fresh, cooked or brewed into a 'tea'. Psilocybin is from the same chemical family as LSD so its effects are similar; it usually takes about 30–50 mushrooms to produce an LSD-like hallucinogenic experience. Physical effects of psilocybin are usually experienced within 20 minutes of ingestion and can last for 6 hours. Other hallucinogens include *Amanita muscaria* (fly agaric mushrooms) and mescaline, which is derived from the peyote cactus. The legal status, sought-after effects and adverse effects are given in Table 13.6.

PCP (phencyclidine)

PCP, a pure white crystalline powder, is most often called 'angel dust'. It was first developed as an anaesthetic in the 1950s but was discontinued for therapeutic use because of its hallucinatory effects. PCP has a distinctive bitter chemical taste and comes in a in a variety of tablets, capsules and colored powders. It can be swallowed, smoked, sniffed or injected. PCP is sometimes sprinkled on cannabis, mint or parsley and smoked. PCP has been sold as mescaline, THC (tetrahyrdrocannabinol) or other psychoactive drugs. Interactions with other central nervous system depressants, such as alcohol and benzodiazepines, can lead to coma. High doses of PCP can also cause seizures, coma and death (though death more often results from accidental injury or suicide during PCP intoxication). The legal status, sought-after effects and adverse effects are presented in Table 13.7.

Table 13.6 Characteristics of psilocybin.

Street names	■ Magic mushroom
Legal status	■ Psilocybin or psilocybin-containing mushrooms ('fungus (of any kind) which contains psilocin or an ester of psilocin') are a class A drug under the Drugs Act 2005 ■ This does not include fly agaric, which is still legal
Sought-after effects	■ The sought-after effects are similar to LSD, but the hallucinogenic trip is often milder and shorter
Adverse effects	■ Small quantities cause relaxation and slight changes in mood ■ Larger quantities can cause stomach pain, nausea and vomiting, diarrhoea, shivering, a numbing of the mouth, muscle weakness, dizziness, drowsiness and panic reactions ■ Higher doses can also cause perceptual changes, distortion of body image and hallucinations ■ Some people eat poisonous mushrooms thinking they are mushrooms containing psilocybin. This can be very dangerous as some poisonous mushrooms can cause death or permanent liver damage within hours of ingestion ■ Fly agaric mushrooms often cause nausea and stomach pain ■ Tolerance builds up with use of mushrooms in so far as the user needs to space out 'trips' to get the desired effects

Dependence and tolerance

PCP causes the development of tolerance and strong psychological dependence. Repeated abuse can lead to craving and compulsive PCP-seeking behavior. Recent research suggests that repeated or prolonged use of PCP can cause a withdrawal syndrome when drug use is stopped. Symptoms such as memory loss and depression may persist for as long as a year after a chronic user stops taking PCP.

Hypnosedatives

The hypnosedatives include both hypnotics and minor tranquillisers. The barbiturates include tuinal, membutal, sodium amytal, phenobarbitone, etc., and minor tranquillisers (benzodiazepines) include valium (diazepam), librium, ativan, mogadon, temazepam, etc. Others in this group include heminevrin, chloral hydrate, etc. Hypnosedatives are drug of misuse, not only among the illicit drug population, but in the population in general. Benzodiazepines are usually taken by mouth but are sometimes ground up and injected. Temazepam is a popular drug of choice to inject along with heroin. The characteristics of this group of drugs are given in Table 13.8.

Table 13.7 Characteristics of PCP.

Street names	■ Angel dust
Legal status	■ PCP is a class A substance in the UK
Sought-after effects	■ The user experiences alterations in thought, mood, sensory perception and body awareness ■ The drug has been known to alter mood states in an unpredictable fashion ■ For some users, PCP in small amounts acts as a stimulant, speeding up bodily functions, and for others it acts as a depressant ■ A drug-taking episode may produce feelings of detachment from reality, including distortions of space, time and body image; another episode may produce hallucinations, panic and fear
Adverse effects	■ The effects of PCP use are unpredictable, can be felt within minutes of ingestion, and can last for many hours ■ Some users report feeling the effects of the drug for a number of days ■ A low to moderate amount of PCP often causes the user to feel detached, distant and estranged from his or her environment ■ Other effects include numbness, slurred speech, loss of coordination, rapid and involuntary eye movements, exaggerated gait, shallow and rapid breathing, increased blood pressure, elevated heart rate and increased temperature ■ Nausea, blurred vision, dizziness and decreased awareness can also occur. High doses of PCP can cause convulsions, coma, hyperthermia and death. Long-term users report memory loss, difficulties with speech and thinking, depression and weight loss ■ A temporary schizophrenic-type psychosis may last for days or weeks. Auditory hallucinations, image distortion, severe mood disorders and amnesia may also occur

Volatile substances

Lighter fuel refills, glues, aerosols, typewriter correction fluids/thinners, dry cleaning fluids, de-greasing compounds, etc. are products that are subjected to misuse. Sniffers of volatile substances heighten the desired effect by increasing the concentration of the vapour and excluding air; for example by sniffing from a bag or by placing a plastic bag over the head while inhalation takes place. Solvent misuse seems to occur in localised areas, for example in a particular housing estate, school or social group. Approximately one in ten secondary school children try sniffing. The peak age of experimentation is approximately 13–14 years. A report (St George's 2007) reveals that in 2005 there were 45 deaths in the

Table 13.8 Characteristics of hypnosedatives.

Street names	▪ Downers, barbs, tranx
Legal status	▪ Benzodiazepines and barbiturates are prescription-only medicines and are class C and B controlled drugs, respectively. It is illegal to supply these psychoactive substances
Therapeutic uses	▪ Barbiturates have been used medically in anaesthesia and in the treatment of epilepsy and, rarely nowadays, insomnia ▪ Minor tranquillisers are often prescribed for the relief of anxiety and stress
Adverse effects	▪ Barbiturates are depressant drugs and their effects are similar to alcohol intoxication ▪ Slurred speech, stumbling, confusion, reduction of inhibition, lowering of anxiety and tension, and impairment of concentration, judgment and performance ▪ The common reactions from minor tranquillisers include fatigue, drowsiness and ataxia. In addition, other effects may include constipation, incontinence, urinary retention, dysarthria, blurred vision, hypotension, nausea, dry mouth, skin rash and tremor. In case of overdose, respiratory failure and death may result if these drugs are mixed with alcohol or with each other ▪ Injecting these drugs is particularly hazardous with an increased risk of overdose, gangrene and abscesses ▪ Barbiturates and minor tranquillisers are highly addictive and withdrawal symptoms include anxiety, headaches, cramps in the abdomen, pains in the limbs and even epileptic fits ▪ Withdrawal of barbiturates can be dangerous and should always be medically supervised

UK associated with volatile substance abuse. This is the lowest annual total recorded since 1980. In 2005, butane from all sources accounted for 36 of the 45 deaths, and of these butane cigarette lighter refills formed the largest group.

Many young people who sniff these substances have accidents while they are intoxicated and suffer serious health consequences. Some users go on to become heavy and frequent solvent misusers. The pattern of use includes children from all areas and social classes and both genders. There is some evidence that girls are less likely to become chronic users and prevalence is higher in inner city areas. The street names, legal status, sought-after effects and short-term and long-term effects are presented in Table 13.9.

The inhaled solvent vapours are absorbed quickly through the lungs and rapidly reach the brain. Part of the effect is the reduction in oxygen intake. Respiratory rate and heart rate are depressed and repeated or deep inhalation can result in an 'overdose', causing disorientation, loss of control and unconsciousness. The effects appear quickly and disappear, usually less than 45 minutes after sniffing has stopped. There may be a hangover effect with headache and poor concentration

Table 13.9 Characteristics of volatile substances.

Street names	▓ Solvents, inhalants, glue, gas, thinners, hair sprays, tolly, huff
Legal status	▓ The Intoxicating Substances Supply Act (England and Wales) 1985 makes it an offence to supply a young person under 18 years with a substance which the supplier knows or has reason to believe will be used 'to achieve intoxication' ▓ The law is mainly directed to shopkeepers but could also be applied to anyone who sells or gives a young person a sniffable product ▓ In Scotland, the common law provides for a similar offence of 'recklessly' selling solvents to children knowing they are going to inhale them ▓ An amendment to the Consumer Protection Act (The Cigarette Lighter Refill (Safety) Regulations) 1999 made it an offence to 'supply any cigarette lighter refill canister containing butane or a substance with butane as a constituent part to any person under the age of eighteen years'
Sought-after effects	▓ After inhalation of volatile substances, effects are experienced within a matter of minutes ▓ Users typically experience sensations akin to taking alcohol – being giggly and disorientated, possibly being uncoordinated and feeling dizzy. Nausea is not uncommon
Short-term effects	▓ Depressed respiration rate ▓ Depressed heart rate ▓ Loss of co-ordination ▓ Disorientation ▓ Loss of consciousness ▓ Drowsiness ▓ Hangover ▓ Accidental death ▓ Heart failure
Long-term effects	▓ Damage to brain, kidneys and liver ▓ Exhaustion ▓ Amnesia ▓ Loss of concentration ▓ Weight loss ▓ Depression

for about a day. Chronic misuse of aerosols and cleaning fluids can cause renal and hepatic damage, a lack of ability to control movement, weight loss, depression and tremor. These symptoms usually clear when sniffing ceases. Tolerance can develop but physical dependence does not constitute a significant problem. Psychological dependence occurs in susceptible youngsters with concomitant family or personality problems. These individuals are also more prone to become 'lone sniffers' instead of the usual pattern of sniffing in groups.

Table 13.10 Characteristics of over-the-counter drugs.

Legal status	▦ No prescriptions are required to purchase these substances
Therapeutic uses	▦ Many of these medical preparations are used for the relief of pain, coughs, the common cold, treatment of diarrhoea and respiratory conditions
Effects	▦ Some of these substances are taken in large doses and are often combined with other drugs to obtain the desired effects
	▦ Antihistamines may be used for their sedative value and/or mixed with methadone or heroin
	▦ The amphetamine derivatives in decongestants may be used as a stimulant; cough linctuses and diarrhoea drug treatments may be used for their opiate content

Over-the-counter drugs

Several medicinal preparations are available without prescription and are sold in chemist shops and are purchased for their non-medical therapeutic effects. These are depressants such as codeine linctus, Colles Browne's mixture, Gee's Linctus and kaolin and morphine. Stimulants include Fenox, Mercocaine, lozenges, Sinutads, Sudafed and Do-Do. Travel sickness pills such as Kwells containing hallucinogenic compounds are also available over-the-counter. The characteristics of over-the-counter drugs are given in Table 13.10.

Smart and eco drugs

Smart drugs, smart products and eco drugs are new substances that are composed of multiple ingredients. Smart drugs are referred to as substances taken with the purpose of enhancing cognitive functions and may have stimulating, sedating or hallucinogenic effects. They are promoted as mind enhancers, mind boosters, brain boosters, intelligence boosters and are considered to be safe, healthy and harmless substitutes for illicit drugs. Some of the smart drugs are reported to enhance sexual behaviour, physical endurance, muscle power and emotional intelligence.

Cognitive enhancers have been used to treat people with neurological or mental disorders, but there are a growing number of healthy individuals who use these substances in the hope of getting smarter. These substances are classified as:

▦ Smart drugs: improving cognitive functions.
▦ Smart drinks and nutrients.
▦ Smart products: herbal mixtures and food additives. These mimic the effects of illicit drug such as ecstasy.
▦ Eco drugs: herbs, plants and mixtures of both. Some hallucinogenic or euphoric effects are linked with their use.
▦ Energising drinks: high caffeine content with guarana and taurine.

Their effects can vary considerably. Some smart products are highly stimulating, and others induce a mild form of excitement and/or euphoria. Eco drugs, such as hallucinogenic mushrooms, Kava Kava and Yohimbe are vegetable substances that can produce a psychotropic or physical effect. It is not always clear which laws and regulations apply to these substances. In addition, there is limited evidence about the effects of these substances and the risks involved in using these substances.

Summary of key points

- LSD is an odourless, colourless and tasteless powder. LSD can be swallowed, sniffed, injected or smoked.
- The effects of LSD may cause panic, confusion, impulsive behaviour, unpleasant illusions (bad trip) and flashbacks and may precipitate psychotic reactions.
- GHB causes intoxication resembling alcohol or ketamine intoxication and can lead to respiratory depression and death, especially when combined with alcohol.
- At high doses of GHB, convulsions, coma and respiratory collapse can occur.
- Most deaths have occurred when GHB was taken with alcohol or other drugs.
- Withdrawal from GHB may cause symptoms similar to acute withdrawal from alcohol or barbiturates (delirium tremens) and can cause convulsions, paranoia and hallucinations.
- Some ketamine users' experiences involve a terrifying feeling of almost complete sensory detachment that is likened to a near-death experience.
- With very high doses of ketamine, coma and severe hypertension may occur; deaths are unusual.
- It usually takes about 30–50 mushrooms containing psilocybin to produce a hallucinogenic experience, similar to that experienced with LSD.
- Higher doses of psilocybin cause perceptual changes, distortion of body image and hallucinations.
- Some people eat poisonous mushrooms thinking they are mushrooms containing psilocybin.
- High doses of PCP can cause convulsions, coma, hyperthermia and death.
- Long-term users of PCP report memory loss, difficulties with speech and thinking, depression and weight loss.
- Recent research suggests that repeated or prolonged use of PCP can cause a withdrawal syndrome when drug use is stopped.
- Hypnosedatives are drug of misuse not only among the illicit drug population but in the population in general.
- Benzodiazepines and barbiturates are prescription-only medicines and are class C and B controlled drugs, respectively.
- Barbiturates are depressant drugs and their effects are similar to alcohol intoxication.
- Some organic-based substances produce effects similar to alcohol or anaesthetics when their vapours are inhaled.
- After inhalation of volatile substances, effects are experienced within a matter of minutes.
- Over-the-counter drugs are taken in large doses and are often combined with other drugs to obtain the desired effects.
- The amphetamine derivatives in decongestants may be used as a stimulant; cough linctuses and diarrhoea drug treatments may be used for their opiate content.
- Smart drugs are substances taken with the purpose of enhancing cognitive functions and may have stimulating, sedating or hallucinogenic effects.

References

DrugScope (2009) *DrugScope highlights concerns over trends in ketamine use.* http://www.drugscope.org.uk/ourwork/pressoffice/pressreleases/DS_concern_ketamine_trends.htm.

Home Office (2008) *Drug Misuse Declared: findings from the British Crime Survey 07/08.* Home Office, London: http://www.homeoffice.gov.uk/rds/pdfs08/hosb1308.pdf.

Home Office (2009) *Drug Misuse Declared: findings from the 2008/09 British Crime Survey. England and Wales.* Home Office Statistical Bulletin. Home Office, London: http://www.homeoffice.gov.uk/rds/pdfs09/hosb1209.pdf.

St George's (2007) *Trends in Death Associated with Abuse of Volatile Substances 1971–2005.* Division of Community Health Sciences Report No. 20. St George's, University of London, London.

14 Nursing Emergencies and Care in Addiction

The use of a combination of alcohol with other psychoactive drug increases the risk of death by overdose and can have serious long-term consequences. Intoxication is a state when there is an intake or more than the normal amount of a psychoactive substance, which produces behavioural or physical changes. An overdose is the accidental or intentional use of a psychoactive substance that exceeds the individual's tolerance. Emergency medical attention is often required by those misusing psychoactive substances as a result of:

- Toxic or adverse effects of the substance.
- The route of administration (injecting may lead to blood poisoning and deep vein thrombosis).
- Lifestyle behaviours (poor malnutrition, dehydration).
- Risk taking whilst under the influence of psychoactive substances (accidents, self-harm).

This chapter covers the two main risks of taking psychoactive substances: intoxication and overdose.

Acute intoxication

Acute intoxication frequently occurs in persons who have more persistent alcohol- or drug-related problems. It is a transient condition following the administration of alcohol or other psychoactive substance, resulting in disturbances in level of consciousness, cognition, perception, affect or behaviour, or other psychophysiological functions and responses (WHO 2005). Intoxication is highly dependent on the type and dose of drug and is influenced by an individual's level of tolerance and other factors. Acute intoxication is the term used in the World Health Organization (WHO) International Classification of Diseases 10 (ICD-10) for intoxication of clinical significance. Acute intoxication is usually closely related to dose levels and the intensity of intoxication lessens with time, and effects eventually disappear in the absence of further use of the psychoactive substance. The symptoms of intoxication do not always reflect the desired or expected effects of the psychoactive substance. The unexpected effects of psychoactive substances are presented in Table 14.1.

Many psychoactive substances are capable of producing different types of effect at different levels. For example, alcohol may have apparently stimulant effects on behaviour at lower dose levels, then may lead to agitation and aggression with increasing dose levels, and produce clear sedation at very high levels. The cultural and personal expectations regarding the effects of the drug will also influence the level of intoxication. The common features of psychoactive intoxication include disinhibition, euphoria, lack of coordination, risk of harm and impaired judgment. However, it is important to recognise the symptoms of alcohol or drug intoxication not only to confirm the presence and severity of the effects of psychoactive substance(s), but also to be able to differentiate the symptoms from other conditions.

Table 14.1 Unexpected effects of psychoactive substances.

Psychoactive drug	Symptoms of intoxication
Alcohol	Agitation Hyperactivity
GHB (gammahydroxybutyrate)	Agitation Hyperactivity
Amphetamine and cocaine	Socially withdrawn Introverted behaviour
Cannabis and hallucinogens	Unpredictable

Risks of alcohol and drug intoxication

Individual in an acute stage of intoxication of alcohol or drugs is most frequently seen in accident and emergency (A&E) departments. Alcohol intoxication rarely requires treatment but it may precipitate seizures by lowering the seizure threshold level. Complications may include trauma, inhalation of vomit, delirium, coma and convulsions, depending on the substance and method of administration. It is extremely common for an intoxicated individual to vomit once or twice.

However, continued vomiting may be a sign of head injury or other serious illness. Trauma and head injuries, caused by poor coordination and judgment when intoxicated, are common. Head injury also increases the risk of seizures. It is possible for an individual who has acute alcohol poisoning to go into respiratory arrest while they are asleep and they can also choke to death on their vomit. Hypothermia is also a high risk factor for homeless problem drinkers. The individual may become belligerent, paranoid and even violent, necessitating the risk of caution and sensitivity when approaching them.

Nursing interventions in acute intoxication

Nursing interventions are based on the urgency and seriousness of the individual with acute intoxication. When an individual is acutely intoxicated, first aid procedures are implemented in relation to:

- A: airway.
- B: breathing.
- C: circulation/cardiac.

The nursing interventions required for an individual with acute intoxication are presented in Table 14.2.

Overdose of psychoactive substances

There has been concern about the high prevalence of mortality amongst substance misusers. The Advisory Council on the Misuse of Drugs (ACMD 2000) report *Reducing Drug-related Deaths* highlighted their concern about this issue and acknowledged that the prevention of drug-related deaths is a matter of pressing urgency. The report indicated that the number of such deaths must be substantially reduced. A higher profile has been highlighted for a range of harm reduction measures to reduce premature death amongst drug users associated with fatal and non-fatal overdoses (Home Office 2002).

An overdose is 'an event in which a person intentionally or accidentally ingests one or more psychoactive substances at unsafe levels, leading to physical trauma, which may require immediate medical care to reverse and manage symptoms and

Table 14.2 Nursing interventions in acute intoxication.

Medical/physical interventions	Psychosocial interventions
Place in recovery position, if appropriate	Orientation
Assessment of airway, breathing and circulation	'Being there'
	Non-judgmental approach in interactions
Assess level of consciousness (Glasgow Coma Scale)	Create a supportive environment
	Assess for risk behaviours (self-harm, potential for violence)
Monitor vital signs	
Implement seizure safety precautions	Contact relatives/friends who are best able to support and reassure the patient
Monitor fluid intake and output	Harm reduction
Implement interventions to decrease systemic absorption of drugs (use of absorbents (e.g. activated charcoal), induced diarrhoea, induced vomiting, gastric lavage) if appropriate	
Monitoring of the withdrawal syndrome	
Administration of antidote, if appropriate	

Source: adapted from Rassool G.H. (2009) *Alcohol and Drug Misuse. A handbook for student and health professionals*, p. 391. Routledge, Oxford. Reproduced with kind permission of Taylor & Francis.

other complications' (NTA 2002: 156). Drug overdose is the most common method of suicide amongst substance misusers and the likelihood of overdose is increased when drugs are taken by injection, and fatal overdose (immediate death) is particularly associated with injecting opioid users (Oyefeso *et al.* 1999).

There is evidence to suggest that about 80% of people who present to A&E departments following self-harm will have taken an overdose of prescribed or over-the-counter medication and most will meet criteria for one or more psychiatric diagnoses at the time they are assessed (Horrocks *et al.* 2003). There are several risk factors that are reported to be associated with an increased likelihood of overdose (Table 14.3).

Nursing interventions in drug overdose

There are some general principles that define nursing interventions of individuals with drug overdose and in any settings emergency treatment should begin immediately. The priority is treating life-threatening problems such as respiratory depression, airway obstruction, cardiovascular collapse and convulsions (epileptic-form seizures) alongside specific measures to treat the overdose. After stabilising the patient, a through history and physical examination are completed.

An alcohol or drug history is taken: obtain information about the substance/s taken, route of administration, amount taken, when and over what period of time. If the individual is unable to participate in the assessment process, collateral

Table 14.3 Predictors of risk associated with overdose.

▨ Injecting drugs (heroin users, high level of dependence)
▨ Poly-drug use (combinations of drugs such as heroin, methadone, alcohol and benzodiazepines)
▨ Concomitant use of other depressant drugs
▨ High tolerance levels (users who have experienced non-fatal overdoses recently)
▨ Low tolerance levels (using opiates when tolerance is low, particularly after a break in use following imprisonment or detoxification)
▨ Cocaine and crack – the use of these drugs among heroin users can play a role in fatal overdoses as they can temporarily mask the sedative effects of heroin and other depressant-type drugs
▨ Poor mental health, depression, hopelessness and suicidal thoughts
▨ Not being in treatment (heroin injectors not in methadone treatment are around four times more likely to die in comparison to those in treatment)
▨ Premature termination of treatment (loss of tolerance, increased poly-drug use after detoxification)
▨ Solitary alcohol or drug use (using drugs alone, especially injecting, places a person at increased risk)
▨ Possibly unexpected changes in purity

Source: adapted from Roberts L. & McVeigh J. (2004) *Lifeguard: act fast save a life. An evaluation of a multi-component information campaign targeted at reducing drug-related deaths in Cheshire and Merseyside*. Centre for Public Health, Faculty of Health and Applied Social Sciences, Liverpool John Moores University, Liverpool.

information should be obtained whenever possible from family members or significant others or past medical notes. Investigations for routine blood count and chemistry, urinalysis and toxicological screens of blood and urine will provide further evidence about the overdose. The level of consciousness should be checked and should continue to be monitored at 15 minute intervals using the Glasgow Coma Scale (Teasdale & Jennett 1974). The nursing interventions with overdose are presented in Table 14.4.

Once the overdose has been treated it is important to assess for depression or self-harm and explore the withdrawal management and treatment intervention options. It is also a good opportunity to discuss harm reduction interventions and to provide health information and information related to specialist alcohol and drug services. Referral to specialist alcohol and drug services is part of the process.

Opiate overdose

Opiate users are prone to accidental overdose because they often overestimate their own tolerance or are unaware of the potency of the drug they use. Most opiate overdoses occur over a 3 hour period after intial drug ingestion (Darke & Zador 1996). The presenting features and nursing interventions of opiate overdose are presented in Table 14.5.

Table 14.4 Nursing interventions with overdose.

▩ Establish a patent airway
▩ Provide ventilation support (artificial respiration, respirator)
▩ Maintain adequate circulatory status (chest compressions, defibrillator, intravenous line)
▩ Control seizures (safety measures, intravenous diazepam)
▩ Administration of drug, if appropriate (e.g. for an opiate overdose, give naloxone)
▩ Monitor vital signs including temperature
▩ Perform an electrocardiogram (EEG) and continue to monitor
▩ Check the level of consciousness; continue to monitor at 15 minute intervals using the Glasgow Coma Scale (Teasdale & Jennett 1974)
▩ Maintain hydration and monitoring of fluid intake and output
▩ Safety precautions must be maintained during acute interventions as the individual may show signs of varying level of consciousness, hallucinations and seizures
▩ Measures to decrease systemic absorption of the substance such as gastric lavage, induced emesis (vomiting), absorbents (activated charcoal) or induced diarrhoea (magnesium) should be used as appropriate
▩ An antidote may be administered depending upon the type of psychoactive substance used
▩ Reassurance and support should be provided

Source: adapted from Rassool G.H. (2009) *Alcohol and Drug Misuse. A handbook for student and health professionals*, p. 394. Routledge, Oxford. Reproduced with kind permission of Taylor & Francis.

Table 14.5 Nursing interventions with opiate overdose.

Presenting features	Nursing interventions
Slow respiration (2–7 breaths/minute), usually deep compared with the shallow and more rapid respiration associated with intoxication by barbiturates, etc. Pinpoint pupils Weak pulse Cyanosis Possible pulmonary oedema Twitching of muscles Subnormal temperature may occur	Establish a clear airway Adequate ventilation Oxygenation (if consciousness is impaired) Give oral activated charcoal, provided that the airway can be protected, if a substantial amount has been ingested within 2 hours Administration of naloxone 0.8–2 mg Observe for central nervous system and respiratory depression

The pharmacological treatment of overdose from opiates is the antidote naloxone hydrochloride (naloxone). A dose of 0.8–2 mg by intravenous injection should be administered, repeated at intervals of 2–3 minutes, to a maximum dose of 10 mg. If respiratory function does not improve, other diagnostic options – such as intoxication with other drugs or other organic causes of loss of consciousness, including hypoglycaemia – should be considered (Department of Health 1999).

If an intravenous route is not accessible due to vein collapse, subcutaneous or intramuscular injection routes should be used. Naloxone is short acting, so repeated injections or intravenous infusion may be needed if a longer acting opiate such as methadone has been taken. Naloxone can be given as a continuous intravenous infusion of 2 mg diluted in 500 ml of an intravenous solution titrated at a rate determined by the clinical response (Department of Health 1999). In methadone overdose, the effects can persist for up to 72 hours. Even in circumstances where patients have been resuscitated, depending on the magnitude of the overdose, they should be observed as an in-patient for a period of up to 72 hours. For high-dose intoxication, naloxone infusion should be considered.

Cocaine overdose

Excessive doses, whether snorted, injected or smoked, can lead to overdose and sudden death from respiratory or heart failure. Cocaine-related deaths are often a result of cardiac arrest or seizures followed by respiratory arrest. In pregnant women, it can have devastating effects on the fetus, producing congenital abnormalities, or it can induce spontaneous abortion. The physical symptoms of cocaine overdose may include chest pain, nausea, blurred vision, fever, muscle spasms, convulsions and coma. Hyperthermia (elevated body temperature) and convulsions occur with cocaine overdoses, and if not treated immediately, can result in death.

Ecstasy overdose

Overdose from ecstasy is usually characterised by very high body temperature and blood pressure, hallucinations and an elevated heart beat. This is especially dangerous for those who have an existing cardiovascular problem, and for people with depression or other psychological disorders. Sudden death through overheating, dehydration, heavy alcohol consumption or drinking too much water has led to collapse, convulsions or renal failure. However, drinking too much water in an attempt to stay 'safe' is more dangerous. The excess water (dilutional hyponatraemia) causes the brain to swell inside the skull, which puts pressure on the brainstem and can lead to coma and death. In relation to harm reduction, it is advised that the wearing of light, loose clothing, drinking plenty of non-alcoholic fluids as well as stopping dancing when feeling exhausted, could help reduce the possible complications of the drug. About ten ecstasy-related deaths have been reported in the UK each year for the past several years.

Amyl nitrite overdose

Overdose from amyl nitrite includes the symptoms of nausea, vomiting, hypotension, hypoventilation, shortness of breath and fainting.

GHB overdose

Overdosing can lead to a loss of consciousness and coma. It is not recommended that asthmatics or those with any form of respiratory or low blood pressure disorder take this drug. Most deaths have occurred when GHB (gammahydroxybutyrate) was taken with alcohol or other drugs. When taken in combination with other psychoactive substances, the effects of GHB are more intense and the risk of toxic effects and overdose increases.

Overdose of GHB can be difficult to treat because of its multiple effects on the body. GHB overdose often causes life-threatening respiratory depression, bradycardia and consequent heart failure. GHB tends to cause nausea and vomiting, particularly when combined with alcohol and the most likely risk of death from GHB overdose is inhalation of vomit while unconscious.

Ketamine overdose

With large or repeat doses hallucinations occur, for example loss of sense of time, feeling disconnected from the body and near-death experiences. A few deaths have occurred from overdose through heart or respiratory failure.

Volatile substance overdose

Volatile solvent overdose is rare. The toxicity of volatile substances varies greatly, depending on the substance. Generally, signs are cardiac arrhythmias, hypoxia and neurological impairment. However, there is considerable risk of accidental injury or death if the individual becomes intoxicated in a hazardous environment. During vomiting there is the risk of choking if the snuffer has been intoxicated to the point of unconsciousness. If a plastic bag has been placed over the head in order to assist inhalation of the substance, suffocation becomes a real risk. Some volatile substances such as aerosol gases and cleaning fluids can sensitise the heart, causing heart failure. Some gases squirted directly into the mouth can cause death from suffocation. Sniffing from small bags held to the mouth or nose has caused fewer deaths than the practice of inhaling butane and similar gases with plastic bags placed over the head.

Overdose with other drugs

No antidote exists for the treatment of overdose from other psychoactive substances such as amphetamines, cocaine, cannabis, LSD (lysergic acid diethylamide), ecstasy, barbiturates and alcohol. In such overdoses, respiration must be maintained by artificial means until the drugs are removed from the system. Some drugs may help speed the excretion of barbiturates. The use of tricyclic antidepressants is common with substance misusers. Antidepressants in large dosage can cause coma, cardiac arrhythmias and anticholinergic effects and mortality risk is high. For cocaine overdose, diazepam (Valium) is recommended for the agitation, irritability, seizures and hyperexcitable state. This also helps control the rapid heart rate and elevated blood pressure. Nursing interventions should therefore be aimed at the presenting symptoms and may include:

- Management of the unconscious patient.
- Management of hypothermia.
- Management of acute psychosis.

Summary of key points

- Intoxication and overdose are the potential consequences of substance misuse, whether the psychoactive substance is illicit, prescribed or over-the-counter.
- Acute intoxication frequently occurs in persons who have more persistent alcohol- or drug-related problems.
- The type and dose of drug and the individual's level of tolerance have a significant influence on the state of intoxication.
- Drug-related deaths are deaths where the underlying cause is poisoning, drug misuse or addiction.
- Drug overdose is the most common method of suicide amongst substance misusers and the likelihood of overdose is increased when drugs are taken by injection.
- Fatal overdose (immediate death) is particularly associated with injecting opioid users.
- Overdose amongst substance misusers is an acute life-threatening emergency.
- The treatment of overdose from opiates is the antidote naloxone.
- No antidote exists for the treatment of overdose from other drugs such as amphetamines, cocaine, cannabis, LSD, ecstasy, barbiturates and alcohol.

References

ACMD (Advisory Council on the Misuse of Drugs) (2000) *Reducing Drug-related Deaths. A report by the Advisory Council on the Misuse of Drugs*. The Stationery Office, London.

Darke S. & Zador D. (1996) Fatal heroin 'overdose': a review. *Addiction*, 91(12), 1765–1772.

Department of Health (1999) *Drug Misuse and Dependence – guidelines on clinical management*. The Stationery Office, London.

Home Office (2002) *Updated Strategy 2002*. Home Office, London: www.drugs.gov.uk.

Horrocks J., Price S., House A. & Owens D. (2003) Self-injury attendances in the accident and emergency department. *British Journal of Psychiatry*, 183(1), 34–39.

NTA (National Treatment Agency) (2002) *Models of Care for Treatment of Adult Drug Misusers. Parts 1 and 2*. NTA Publications, London.

Oyefeso A., Ghodse A.H., Clancy C. & Corkery J.M. (1999) Suicide among drug addicts in the UK. *British Journal of Psychiatry*, 175(3), 277–282.

Rassool, G.H. (2009) *Alcohol and Drug Misuse. A handbook for student and health professionals.* Routledge, Oxford.

Roberts L. & McVeigh J. (2004) *Lifeguard: act fast save a life. An evaluation of a multi-component information campaign targeted at reducing drug-related deaths in Cheshire and Merseyside.* Centre for Public Health, Faculty of Health and Applied Social Sciences, Liverpool John Moores University, Liverpool.

Teasdale G. & Jennett B. (1974) Assessment of coma and impaired consciousness. A practical scale. *Lancet*, 2(7872), 81–84.

WHO (World Health Organization) (2005) *The ICD-10 Classification of Mental and Behavioural Disorders: diagnostic criteria for research.* WHO, Geneva.

15 Blood-Borne Viruses

Blood-borne infection is transmitted by infected blood or blood-stained body fluids coming into contact with an open lesion on the skin and by injury with a sharp object contaminated with infected blood. However, the risk of transmission of blood-borne viruses depends on a number of factors including:

- The frequency and scale of contact with blood and body fluids.
- The behaviour of different persons.
- The type of material contact is made with.
- The infectious nature of the person/material.

The major risks posed to people who inject illicit drugs are the human immuno-deficiency virus (HIV) and hepatitis viruses B and C (HBV, HCV). This is largely because of transfer of blood through the sharing of contaminated injecting equipment or of environmental contamination in injecting settings. In England, *The National Strategy on Sexual Health and HIV* (Department of Health 2001) covers a wide sexual health agenda, including HIV, sexually transmitted infections (STIs) and unintended pregnancies in the areas of prevention, testing, treatment and care, stigma and discrimination. In relation to HIV and STIs, the Strategy aims to:

Addiction for Nurses By G. Hussein Rassool. © 2010 G. Hussein Rassool

■ Reduce the transmission of HIV and STIs.
■ Reduce the prevalence of undiagnosed HIV and STIs.
■ Improve health and social care for people living with HIV.
■ Reduce the stigma associated with HIV and STIs.

Fear and prejudice regarding blood-borne viruses, particularly HIV-infected individuals, remains an issue in most societies. There have been incidences of violence towards people with HIV infection and their property, as well as stigmatisation by friends, family, neighbours and colleagues. Stigma and discrimination can impede disclosure and deter people from working and using health care and social care services, thereby contributing to the social exclusion of people living with HIV (Department of Health 2007).

Human immunodeficiency virus

HIV is the virus that causes AIDS (acquired immune deficiency syndrome). AIDS is a collection of rare infections and cancers that people with HIV can develop. A person is diagnosed with AIDS when he or she has less than 200 CD4 cells/mm^3 and/or one of 21 AIDS-defining opportunistic infections. Blood, blood products, semen, vaginal secretions, donor organs and tissues, and breast milk have been implicated in the transmission of infection. Most HIV transmission occurs as a result of:

■ Unprotected vaginal or anal intercourse.
■ Sharing contaminated needles and syringes.
■ Transfusion of contaminated blood and blood products.
■ Transmission from mother to baby *in utero*, at birth or via breast feeding.

AIDS is among the leading causes of death globally and remains the primary cause of death in Africa. However, new data show that global HIV prevalence (the percentage of people living with HIV) has levelled off and that the number of new infections has fallen, in part as a result of the impact of HIV programmes (UNAIDS & WHO 2007). The number of people dying from AIDS-related illnesses has declined in the last 2 years, due in part to the life-prolonging effects of antiretroviral therapy. There is concern regarding the steady increase in heterosexual HIV transmission, especially in the black ethnic minority, and transmission of HIV among injecting drug users. A survey found that one in three people living with HIV in the UK do not know that they are infected and that there is still stigma attached to being tested for HIV (National AIDS Trust 2007a). People are also less aware of the risks of HIV transmission than they were 10 years ago. In addition, the survey found that one in five people were not aware of the risk of HIV infection through sex without a condom, the most common route of transmission in the UK. Some of the opportunistic infections and tumours in late stage of AIDS are presented in Table 15.1.

Table 15.1 Opportunistic infections and tumours in the late stage of AIDS.

Bacterial	Viral	Fungal	Protozoal	Tumour
Mycobacterial tuberculosis	Papovaviruses	*Candida*	*Pneumocystis carinii*	Kaposi's sarcoma
Mycobacterium avium complex	Cytomegalovirus	*Cryptococcus*	Toxoplasmosis	Non-Hodgkin's lymphoma
Salmonella	Herpes (simplex and zoster)	*Aspergillus*	*Cryptosporidium*	
Shigella			*Isospora*	Cervical cancer

Testing and counselling

In order to ascertain whether an individual is infected with HIV, an HIV antibody test or HIV test is undertaken. The standard HIV test looks for antibodies in a person's blood. Babies retain their mother's antibodies for up to 18 months and may test positive on an HIV antibody test, even if they are actually HIV negative. Most individuals will develop detectable HIV antibodies within 6–12 weeks of infection but may take up to 6 months in very rare cases. If a test is taken earlier than 3 months, this may result in an unclear test result as an infected person may not yet have developed antibodies to HIV. All women in England are now offered and recommended an HIV test as part of their antenatal care, not just those in high prevalence areas. The early detection of HIV infection allows women who may have been infected to seek advice and make decisions about conception, the management of their pregnancy and breast feeding.

The UK Health Departments recommend that named testing for evidence of HIV infection should only be undertaken with informed consent, individuals having received information about how HIV is transmitted, the significance of both positive and negative results and a discussion of the particular needs and interests relevant to the individual. Key components of the pre-test discussion and post-test counselling are presented in Table 15.2.

Prevention and treatment

HIV can be transmitted in three main ways: sexual transmission, transmission through blood and mother-to-child transmission. Sexual behaviour is a major factor determining the transmission of HIV. Some groups need targeted sexual health information and HIV/STI prevention strategies because they are at higher risk, are particularly vulnerable or have particular access requirements (Department of Health 2001). Higher risk groups include young people (in or out of care), gay and bisexual men, injecting drug misusers, adults and children living with HIV-infected people, sex workers and people in prisons. The report

Table 15.2 Pre-test discussion and post-test counseling in HIV.

Pre-test content	Discussion
Nature of HIV	▩ Modes of transmission ▩ Difference between HIV and AIDS ▩ Methods to reduce transmission ▩ Provision of materials about risk reduction strategies
Risk activities/need for test	▩ Unsafe sexual practices ▩ History of drug use ▩ Injecting behaviour ▩ History of exposure to blood/blood products ▩ Tattooing ▩ Occupational risk ▩ Overseas travel with exposure to high-risk activities
Advantages of testing	▩ Allows an individual to form strategies to protect sexual partners ▩ Allow interventions to reduce vertical transmission (pregnant women) ▩ Allows for appropriate medical care ▩ Allows effective prophylactic care ▩ Allows decisions for future plans ▩ Reduction of needless anxiety about HIV infection
Disadvantages of testing	▩ Psychological complications ▩ Possible adverse impact on relationships (family, partners, work) ▩ Possible restrictions such as travelling abroad
Test procedure and result giving	▩ Positive, negative and indeterminate results
Obtaining informed consent	▩ Written note
Post-test counselling	**If HIV positive**
▩ Address immediate concerns ▩ Provide support for those who are positive ▩ Provide information on prevention of HIV transmission	▩ Address patient's immediate reactions ▩ Refer for specialist management and treatment ▩ Give details of support service ▩ Offer follow-up appointments ▩ Ongoing support (legal issues, support for carers and partners, etc.)

Source: adapted from EAGA (Expert Advisory Group on AIDS) (2002) *HIV Testing: guidelines for pre-test discussion.* Department of Health, London. Rassool G.H. (2009) *Alcohol and Drug Misuse. A handbook for student and health professionals,* p. 181. Routledge, Oxford. Reproduced with kind permission of Taylor & Francis.

by the National Aids Trust (2007b) *Commissioning HIV Prevention Activities in England* recommended that greater investment in effective prevention programmes that target high-risk communities, and in particular gay men and black African communities, is needed to tackle the growing HIV epidemic in the UK.

Antiretroviral treatment for HIV infection consists of drugs that work against HIV infection itself by slowing down replication of HIV in the body. The antiretroviral drugs are usually prescribed in combinations of three or more. This is called combination therapy or highly active antiretroviral therapy (HAART). HAART has been proved effective in controlling HIV and delaying the onset of AIDS for many people. However, the treatments are not effective for everyone and can have adverse effects; for those showing drug resistance to the effects of an antiretroviral drug, another combination therapy has to be taken. Despite this success, the person will still have HIV in their body. Some people with HIV use complementary therapies including vitamin and mineral supplements, herbal remedies, meditation, massage and acupuncture.

Tuberculosis

Tuberculosis (TB) is an infection caused by a bacterium (germ) called Mycobacterium tuberculosis and usually affects the lungs (pulmonary) but any part of the body can be affected. Transmission occurs through coughing infectious droplets, and usually requires prolonged close contact with an infectious case. The typical signs of TB are:

- Chronic or persistent cough.
- Sputum production.
- Fatigue.
- Lack of appetite.
- Weight loss.
- Night sweats.
- Fever.

TB is common in people with AIDS and is one of the leading causes of death in HIV-infected people. As HIV affects the immune system, this increases the likelihood of people acquiring TB infection. HIV infection is the most potent risk factor for converting latent TB into active TB, while TB bacteria accelerate the progress of AIDS infection in the patient. The two diseases represent a deadly combination, since they are more destructive together than either disease alone. Furthermore, without proper treatment approximately 90% of those living with HIV die within months of contracting TB. TB is harder to diagnose, progresses faster in HIV-infected people and is almost certain to be fatal if undiagnosed or left untreated. TB is curable with a combination of specific antibiotics, but treatment must be continued for at least 6 months.

Hepatitis C

The major route of hepatitis C transmission in the UK is by sharing equipment for injecting drug use, mainly via blood-contaminated needles and syringes. Mother-to-baby transmission does occur, either *in utero* or at the time of birth, but appears to be uncommon. However, it is advisable to avoid breast feeding. Sexual transmission of hepatitis C is possible but uncommon. There is some evidence that transmission may occur through the sharing of toothbrushes, razors and other personal toiletry items that could be contaminated with blood. Transmission can occur through medical and dental procedures and there is a high risk from tattooing, ear piercing, body piercing and acupuncture with unsterile equipment. The signs and symptoms of the early-stage and later stage of hepatitis C are presented in Table 15.3.

Most people who become infected with hepatitis C are unaware of it at the time because it produces no signs or symptoms during its earliest stages. In many cases, signs and symptoms may not appear for decades, which make the infection difficult to recognise. Some patients will report quite severe symptoms with no clinical signs of liver disease, while cirrhosis can be present without any obvious symptoms. If hepatitis progresses, its symptoms begin to point to the liver as the source of illness and causes jaundice, foul breath, a bitter taste in the mouth and dark or 'tea-colored' urine. Alcohol consumption and co-infection with HIV or hepatitis B are strongly associated with increased likelihood of progression to severe liver complications.

Testing, prevention and harm reduction

Like HIV testing there are clear guidelines on testing and counselling in hepatitis C infection. The guidelines on HIV pre-test discussion and post-test counselling

Table 15.3 Signs and symptoms of hepatitis C.

Early stage	Later stage
Slight fatigue	Fatigue
Nausea	Lack of appetite
Poor appetite	Nausea
Muscle and joint pains	Vomiting
Tenderness (area of the liver)	Pain and discomfort
	Jaundice (yellow skin and eyes)
	High temperature
	Weight loss
	Poor memory
	Anxiety
	Depression
	Alcohol intolerance

Source: adapted from Rassool G.H. (2009) *Alcohol and Drug Misuse. A handbook for student and health professionals*, p. 185. Routledge, Oxford. Reproduced with kind permission of Taylor & Francis.

Table 15.4 Provision of services and harm reduction in hepatitis C.

Service provision	Harm reduction strategies
Provision of needle, syringe and other injecting equipment exchange services in the community	Stop or reduce alcohol consumption
	Not to donate blood
	Carry an organ donor card
Safe disposal of used needles and syringes	Never to share any injecting equipment
Provision of outreach and peer education services	Use condoms to minimise the risk of sexual transmission (although rare)
Provision of specialist drug treatment services	Not to share razors or toothbrushes or any toiletry equipment contaminated with blood
Provision of information and advice about hepatitis C and other blood-borne viruses and the risks of injecting drugs (including stopping injecting, the risks of sharing injecting equipment and avoiding initiating others)	Avoid body piercing
Provision of disinfecting tablets throughout the prison estate	

Source: adapted from Department of Health (2002) *Hepatitis C Strategy for England*. Department of Health, London. Rassool G.H. (2009) *Alcohol and Drug Misuse. A handbook for student and health professionals*, Routledge, Oxford. Reproduced with kind permission of Taylor & Francis.

are applicable for the hepatitis C test. In order to reduce or minimise hepatitis C infections, the Department of Health's (2002) *Hepatitis C Strategy for England* recommended the provision of a number of services (Table 15.4). In addition, all NHS organisations need to reduce the risk of hepatitis C transmission within health care settings by the adoption of rigorous standard (universal) infection control precautions, occupational health checks for staff and effective management of occupational blood exposure incidents. If there is a diagnosis of hepatitis C, harm reduction needs to be discussed with the patient (Table 15.4).

At present there is no vaccination against hepatitis C and those who are hepatitis C positive should have their liver function checked on a regular basis to check for liver damage. The treatment of hepatitis C has improved significantly with the use of two medications. The National Institute for Health and Clinical Excellence (NICE 2009) recommends a combination therapy of peginterferon alfa plus ribavirin in the treatment of mild and chronic hepatitis C. The combination therapy is the treatment of choice and lasts for 6–12 months, and can eliminate the virus in about 50% of people infected.

Hepatitis B

Hepatitis B is a blood-borne viral infection that can be prevented through vaccination. Transmission of hepatitis B usually occurs by:

▣ Unprotected sexual intercourse.
▣ Injecting drug misusers sharing blood-contaminated injecting equipment.
▣ Receipt of contaminated blood or blood products.
▣ From an infected mother to her baby (perinatal).
▣ Child-to-child contact in household settings.
▣ Tattooing and body piercing.

The hepatitis B virus can cause a short-term (acute) infection, which may or may not cause symptoms. Some people may experience sore throat, tiredness, joint pains, nausea and vomiting and a loss of appetite. Acute infection can be severe causing abdominal discomfort and jaundice. Following an acute infection, a minority of infected adults (but most infected babies) develop a persistent infection called chronic hepatitis B. Many people with chronic hepatitis B remain well but become chronic carriers. They are unaware that they are infected but can still pass on the virus to others. These individuals will remain infectious and will be at risk of developing cirrhosis and primary liver cancer.

The most important measure in the protection against hepatitis B is by immunisation, which provides protection in up to 90% of recipients. Hepatitis B vaccination should be carried out as soon after initial presentation as possible in all drug users, regardless of the presence of injecting. The vaccine is given as a series of three intramuscular doses. Alpha interferon is used to treat patients with chronic hepatitis B infection.

Summary of key points

■ Blood-borne viruses, especially HIV, HBV and HCV, pose major risks to the health of people who inject illicit drugs.
■ Most HIV transmission occurs via unprotected vaginal or anal intercourse, sharing contaminated needles and syringes, the transfusion of contaminated blood and blood products. from mother to baby *in utero*, at birth or via breast feeding, or through the transfusion of contaminated blood and blood products.
■ There is concern regarding the steady increase in heterosexual HIV transmission, especially in the black ethnic minority, and transmission of HIV among injecting drug users.
■ Fear and prejudice regarding HIV infection act as a barrier to prevention, treatment and care services for people with, or at risk from, HIV.
■ Antiretroviral treatment has had a huge impact on the lives of people with HIV.
■ TB is common in people with AIDS and is one of the leading causes of death in HIV-infected people.
■ Hepatitis means inflammation of the liver. The main cause of hepatitis is through blood-borne viruses.
■ The major route of hepatitis C transmission in the UK is by sharing equipment for injecting drug use, mainly via blood-contaminated needles and syringes.
■ Many people with chronic hepatitis B remain well but become chronic carriers.
■ Alpha interferon is used to treat patients with chronic hepatitis B infection.

References

Department of Health (2001) *The National Strategy for Sexual Health and HIV*. Department of Health, London.

Department of Health (2002) *Hepatitis C Strategy for England*. Department of Health, London: http://www.publications.doh.gov.uk/cmo/hcvstrategy/hcvstratsum.htm (accessed February 2009).

Department of Health (2007) *Tackling HIV Stigma and Discrimination*. Department of Health Implementation Plan. Department of Health, London: http://www.dh.gov.uk/en/Publicationsandstatistics/Publications/Publications/PolicyAndGuidance/DH_076423.

EAGA (Expert Advisory Group on AIDS) (2002) *HIV Testing: guidelines for pre-test discussion*. Department of Health, London: http://www.advisorybodies.doh.gov.uk/eaga/guidelineshivtestdiscuss.htm.

National Aids Trust (2007a) *Updating Our Strategies. Report of an expert seminar on HIV Testing and Prevention, 22 March 2007*. National Aids Trust, London: http://www.nat.org.uk.

National Aids Trust (2007b) *Commissioning HIV Prevention Activities in England*. National Aids Trust, London: http://www.nat.org.uk.

NICE (National Institute of Health and Clinical Excellence) (2009) *NICE Implementation Uptake Report: drugs used to treat hepatitis C*. NICE, London: http://www.nice.org.uk/media/50B/57/UptakeReportHepC.pdf.

Rassool G.H. (2009) *Alcohol and Drug Misuse. A handbook for student and health professionals*. Routledge, Oxford.

UNAIDS & WHO (World Health Organization) (2007) *The 2007 AIDS Epidemic Update*. WHO, Geneva.

16 Prevention and Harm Reduction in Addiction

In the current climate of alcohol and drug misuse, prevention and harm reduction increasingly form part of the role of the nurse in residential and community settings. Every encounter with a patient affords an opportunity for nurses to transmit knowledge about prevention and harm reduction in relation to tobacco smoking, alcohol, psychoactive drugs and sexual health. Various approaches and strategies have been used to prevent alcohol and drug problems, such as awareness raising programmes, law enforcement approaches (demand and supply prevention), community-based health information, school-based education and harm reduction.

The updated UK government alcohol strategy (Department of Health 2007) sets out clear goals and actions to promote sensible drinking and reduce the harm that alcohol can cause. It specifically focuses on the minority of drinkers who cause the most harm to themselves, their communities and their families. The approach of the Department of Health and National Treatment Agency (2007) has wider

Addiction for Nurses By G. Hussein Rassool. © 2010 G. Hussein Rassool

goals of preventing drug misuse and of encouraging stabilisation in treatment and support for abstinence. In relation to harm reduction, the aim is to reduce the number of drug-related deaths and blood-borne virus infections.

Prevention

In public health, prevention activities have been viewed as existing on three levels: primary, secondary and tertiary. This three-stage model has been modified by the Advisory Council on the Misuse of Drugs (ACMD 1984) on the grounds that it was not comprehensive enough to cover all the elements of prevention policies. The ACMD's approach to prevention is based on meeting two basic criteria: (i) reducing the risk of an individual engaging in substance misuse; and (ii) reducing the harm associated with substance misuse. Prevention, in the context of alcohol and drug misuse, has also been defined as 'measures that prevent or delay the onset of drug use as well as measures that protect against risk and reduce harm associated with drug supply and use' (Loxley *et al.* 2004: xiii). Prevention approaches are typically generic to alcohol and all psychoactive substances and may be adapted to address a specific psychoactive substance.

Primary prevention is a process that includes efforts to reduce the demand and stop the occurrence of illegal drug use, any harmful drinking behaviour or tobacco smoking. For example, primary prevention campaigns seek to discourage any alcohol drinking behaviour among young people and those who are in high-risk groups. The focus of primary prevention should not only be targeted at the non-using population but also to experimental, recreational and dependent users. Certain groups are more vulnerable as regards high-risk behaviour and include binge drinkers, pregnant women, youth offenders, injecting drug users, prisoners, prostitutes and the homeless.

Secondary prevention is the prevention of the sequelae of the misuse of psychoactive substances and aims to limit disability or dysfunction. Examples include the rational use of prescribed medication, health information on safer alcohol and drug use, safer sexual practices, and targeting interventions to current users to ensure that they avoid injecting. The harm reduction approach has been widely implemented as a response to the threat presented by blood-borne viruses such as HIV (human immunodeficiency virus) and hepatitis infections.

The aim of the tertiary level of prevention is to restore the individual to an optimal level of functioning and to prevent relapse. In particular, tertiary prevention includes the engagement of residential and community facilities for those who are seeking help for their alcohol- or drug-related problems. Unlike primary and secondary prevention, tertiary prevention involves actual treatment for the disease and is conducted primarily by specialist substance misuse services.

The focus of preventive interventions for nurses is based on primary and secondary interventions in an approach combining assessment, intervention and evaluation. In a global initiative on primary prevention of substance abuse in several countries (WHO 2007), study findings showed that, overall, positive

Table 16.1 Prevention.

Type of prevention	Explanation	Interventions
Primary prevention	Primary prevention is a process that includes efforts to reduce the demand and stop the occurrence of illegal drug use, any harmful drinking behaviour or tobacco smoking To prevent and reduce the initiation of drug use	The provision of health information/teaching, media campaigns and mobilisation of the community
Secondary prevention	Secondary prevention seeks to reduce and limit further health and social harms done by the use and misuse of psychoactive substances through early recognition, intervention and rehabilitation	Rational use of prescribed medication Health information on safer alcohol and drug use and safer sexual practices Harm reduction approach
Tertiary prevention	Tertiary prevention seeks to limit and reduce further complications or dysfunctions through effective care, treatment and rehabilitation services	Management and treatment in specialist alcohol and drug services

outcomes were achieved. Where psychoactive substance use among young people did not (markedly) decrease, the age of onset of psychoactive substance use rose. In certain demographic/age groups, psychoactive substance use remained stable and/or decreased. A summary of the three types of prevention is presented in Table 16.1.

Framework for classifying prevention

An increasingly popular way of classifying prevention initiatives are the universal, selective and indicated prevention programmes (Mrazek & Haggerty 1994). According to this framework, the approaches used in any prevention strategy will depend on the specific aims and intended audience or targeted behaviour/contexts. These strategies focus on different populations and the type of prevention activities are delivered to the specific group. Strategies that aim to inform the broad community about drug use and drug risks are likely to be distinguished from strategies that are aimed at preventing use among school-aged children, and strategies that aim to reduce the problems arising from injecting behaviour (Australian Commonwealth Government 2008). Universal prevention activities may include school-based prevention programmes or mass media campaigns, or they may target whole communities, or parents and families whilst focusing on children and young people.

Table 16.2 An alternative framework of prevention.

	Focus	Target populations	Prevention activities
Universal prevention	The focus of universal programmes is the promotion of health and healthy lifestyles and behaviour and preventing the onset of alcohol and drug use of individual, communities or schools	Targets whole populations at average risk	School-based prevention programmes Mass media campaigns
Selective prevention	Reducing the influence of 'risk factors' and developing resilience (protective factors) Preventing substance use initiation	Targets specific groups at increased average risk	Prevention with high-risk groups Harm Reduction.
Indicated prevention	Problematic drug or alcohol use which requires specialist interventions	Targets individuals with early emerging problems	Harm reduction Pharmacological and psychosocial interventions

Selective prevention programmes target groups or subsets of the population who may have already started to use drugs and/or are at an increased risk of developing substance use problems compared to the general population (Edmonds et al 2005). Prevention programmes are aimed at reducing the influence of 'risk factors', developing resilience (protective factors) and preventing substance use initiation. Indicated prevention programmes (harm reduction) target those exhibiting problematic drug or alcohol use which requires specialist interventions. The framework for classifying prevention initiatives is presented in Table 16.2.

Prevention approaches and interventions

Health education materials may be used to assist in reducing the demand for psychoactive substances through the promotion of healthy lifestyles and suitable alternatives. However, there is also a need to shift substance use education and prevention from its narrow focus of simply providing health information or leaflets to those at risk of alcohol- and drug-related problems to the provision of advice and brief interventions. The most appropriate means of generic and specific interventions to support attitude and behaviour change at population and community levels has peen published by the National Institute of Health and Clinical

Excellence (NICE 2007). The guidance is designed for National Health Service staff and other professionals helping people to change their health-related knowledge, attitudes and behaviour. At community level, primary health care teams are more likely to be involved with preventive health behaviour. However, a workable strategy for nudging the community towards healthier lifestyles and behaviour requires positive partnerships with key agents of change within the community. Table 16.3 summarises the models, goals and interventions of preventive approaches to alcohol and drug use.

The means of implementing prevention strategies include educating young people about the harmful effects of drugs and sexual health education, involving the community in recreational activities, educating the community in stress reduction and coping skills, outreach programmes, harm reduction initiatives and mass media campaigns.

Substance misuse and the workplace

The workplace is an ideal environment for the prevention of the misuse of tobacco smoking, alcohol and drugs. The implementation of health promoting programmes in the workplace has benefited organisations through the reduction of stress, absenteeism and sickness among staff, reductions in staff turnover and increases in organisational efficiency. Nurses have important contributions to make in the development of occupational health services and policy regarding health in the workplace, including substance misuse educational programmes.

During the past two decades, the idea of 'health-promoting hospitals' has been slowly emerging in Europe with its emphasis on health gain through health promotion and disease prevention. A number of initiatives in the creation of health-promoting hospitals are underway and the key principles are derived from the Ottawa Charter for Health Promoting Hospitals (WHO 1992) as a strategic basis. The World Health Organization (WHO 2003) has set five standards describing the principles and actions that should be part of care in every hospital. The five standards address management policy; patient assessment, information and intervention; promoting a healthy workplace; and continuity and cooperation. One of the standards includes health improvement/promotion policies or initiatives that are an integral part of an organisation's quality management system (e.g. their alcohol and drug policy). An alcohol and drug policy is now part of hospital and institutional policies.

Rational use of psychoactive substances

In recent years, there has been an increase in the consumption of psychoactive substances as a consequence of overprescribing and irrational use. This has resulted in increased adverse effects and has produced psychological and physical dependence. Many of the prescribed psychoactive drugs such as hypnotics,

Table 16.3 Prevention approaches to alcohol and drug use.

Approach	Goals	Intervention strategies	Examples
Public health/ medical problems	Reduction of morbidity and mortality	Prevention of ill health Clinical interventions	Early recognition, care, treatment and rehabilitation
Behaviour change	Change of lifestyle and behaviour	Media campaigns Health information on controlled drinking, safer drug use safer sex, and alcohol and driving	Prevent non-smokers starting to smoke Persuade smokers to stop Counselling Harm reduction: reducing or minimising ill effects or harm from alcohol and drugs
Educational	Changing attitudes Increase knowledge and awareness Develop skills in decision making and resilience	Health information on smoking, drinking and drug taking Learning coping skills and stress management	Information about the effects of substance misuse and health-related problems Provision of resources Referral to specialist services
Consumer empowerment	Enabling individuals to identify their health concerns	Advocacy Meeting specific health and socioeconomic needs	Clients identify health needs, types and access to services Community anti-drug campaigns
Social change	Enabling changes to health and social policies Bringing changes to the social environment Improvement in health and social equality in access to services and treatment interventions	Lobbying Political and social actions	Alcohol and drug policy in workplace Limit marketing and advertising of alcohol and tobacco Decriminalisation of drugs Labelling on alcoholic beverages

Source: adapted from Rassool G.H. & Gafoor M. (eds) (1997) *Addiction Nursing – perspectives on professional and clinical practice*. Nelson Thornes, Cheltenham, UK.

sedatives and tranquillisers are frequently the subject of widespread misuse and can result in health-related problems and dependence. With the advent of a self-care approach, consumerism and popular demands for increased self-control have led to the use and misuse of over-the-counter drugs (Rassool 2005). In the context of this chapter, the term rational use means that the right drug is taken by the right patient, in the right dose and for the right duration of therapy, and that the risks of therapy are acceptable (WHO 1989). When the criteria in the process of prescribing are not fulfilled, this is regarded as irrational prescribing.

Many medications contain alcohol, hallucinogenic compounds and narcotics, such as codeine, which can be addictive. The availability and accessibility of medications over the Internet has highlighted the need to be vigilant in public health education as some of the compounds sold may have addictive potential and are life threatening. In 2000, the UK was 19th among the 20 countries with the highest levels of consumption of psychoactive substances for the treatment of moderate to severe pain (INCB 2003). Prescribing and medication management have expanded the role and authority of the nurse. Nurses have a professional responsibility to ensure the rational use of psychoactive drugs. Their knowledge and clinical skills in relation to a wide range of medications and to the sequelae of their misuse can form a basis for effective nursing interventions (Rassool & Winnington 1993). Non-pharmacological therapies such as counselling, relaxation and other therapies may be an alternative to medication with psychoactive substances. It is asserted that while focusing on the misuse of psychoactive drugs, consideration must also be given to the proper use of therapeutic medications (Rassool & Winnington 1993).

Harm reduction approaches

There is now a broad consensus of opinion that recognises that many substance misusers are unable to remain abstinent or lack the readiness to change to be drug-free but nonetheless could benefit from different interventions. Since the mid-1980s, harm reduction is viewed in the UK as an integral and important part of the overall HIV prevention strategy, and a comprehensive and complementary package of interventions for HIV prevention, treatment and care among drug users has been supported.

Harm reduction refers to policies, programmes and practices that aim primarily to reduce the adverse health, social and economic consequences of the use of legal and illegal psychoactive drugs without necessarily reducing drug consumption (IHRA 2009). Harm reduction benefits people who use drugs, their families and the community. Harm reduction means trying to reduce the harm that people do to themselves, or other people, from their substance use. Harm reduction has also been described as a set of practical strategies that reduce the negative consequences of drug use, incorporating a spectrum of strategies from safer use, to managed use to abstinence (Harm Reduction Works 2003). The benefits and limitations of the harm reduction approach are presented in Table 16.4.

Table 16.4 Benefits and limitations of the harm reduction approach.

Advantages	Limitations
A substance misuse-free society is unrealistic	? Provides a disguise for pro-legalisation efforts
It is a pragmatic public health approach	? Encourages illegal use of psychoactive substances
Complements approaches that aim for reductions in drug, alcohol and tobacco consumption	Encourages drinking behaviour
Engages people and motivates them to make contact with substance misuse services	Encourages substance misusers from attaining abstinence
Reduces harm caused by substance misuse	Undercuts abstinence-oriented treatment programmes
Promotes controlled use of psychoactive substances	
Avoids moralistic, stigmatising and judgmental statements about substance misusers	
Reduces accidental death and overdose and saves lives	
Reduces the transmission of blood-borne infections	

Principles of harm reduction

The harm reduction approach to drugs is based on a strong commitment to public health and human rights (IHRA 2009). The principles of harm reduction are outlined in Table 16.5. Hando *et al.* (1999) suggested the following key principles be adopted in designing harm reduction strategies:

- Comprehensive consideration of the full range of social influences and effect of institutions on use.
- Sustainability.
- Clearly targeted, particularly regarding age and stage of drug use.
- Developmentally appropriate and culturally sensitive.
- Based on research knowledge and use of sound methods.
- Clear objectives.
- Aim to reduce risk factors and increase protective factors.
- Evaluation of both positive and negative effects.

An important aspect of harm reduction is its focus on public health, which has improved cooperation between the health, social and criminal justice system and law enforcement agencies. Harm reduction must be carried out in a public health framework and one in which the health, human rights and social needs of drug users, their families and communities are met (Cabinet Office 2005).

Table 16.5 The principles of harm reduction.

■ Accepts that psychoactive substances are a part of our society, and chooses to minimise its harmful effects rather than to ignore or condemn their use

■ Understands that substance misuse is a complex and multifaceted phenomenon that encompasses a continuum of behaviours, ranging from dependence to total abstinence, and acknowledges that some ways of using drugs or alcohol are clearly safer than others

■ Calls for non-judgmental, non-coercive provision of services and resources to individuals who use drugs and the communities in which they live in order to assist them in reducing attendant harm

■ Ensures that substance misusers and those with a history of substance misuse routinely have a real voice in the creation of programmes and policies designed to serve them

■ Affirms substance misusers themselves as the primary agents of reducing the harms of their substance use, and seeks to empower users to share information and support each other in strategies that meet their actual conditions of use

■ Recognises that the realities of poverty, class, racism, social isolation, past trauma, sex-based discrimination and other social inequalities affect both people's vulnerability to and capacity for effectively dealing with substance-related harm

■ Does not attempt to minimize or ignore the real and tragic harm and danger associated with licit and illicit drug use

Source: Harm Reduction Works (2003) *Harm reduction*: www.harmreduction.co.uk/index3.html.

Harm reduction in alcohol

Harm reduction in alcohol can be broadly defined as targeted measures that aim to reduce the negative consequences of drinking rather than focusing on the overall consumption of alcohol (IHRA 2003). Harm reduction offers a pragmatic approach to alcohol consumption and alcohol-related problems based on three core objectives (Marlatt & Witkiewitz 2002):

1 To reduce harmful consequences associated with alcohol use.
2 To provide an alternative to zero tolerance approaches by incorporating drinking goals (abstinence or moderation) that are compatible with the needs of the individual.
3 To promote access to services by offering low-threshold alternatives to traditional alcohol prevention and treatment.

A comprehensive alcohol policy needs population-level interventions that focus on the availability and accessibility of alcohol (such as taxation and restricted licensing hours) and alcohol harm reduction interventions (IHRA 2003). The focus of harm reduction strategies are on particular risk behaviours (such as drinking and driving and binge drinking), special population risk groups (such as pregnant women and young people) and particular drinking contexts (such as bars

Table 16.6 Examples and benefits of the harm reduction approach in alcohol use.

Examples	Benefits
Promoting safer design of drinking environment	Practical approaches
	Realistic approaches
Campaigns against drinking and driving	Not based on national policies,
Serving alcohol in shatter-proof glass to prevent injuries	legislation or funding
	Delivered by local communities based on local needs
Training bar staff to serve alcohol responsibly	Short-term aim to minimise the impacts of alcohol consumption
Minimise violence and antisocial behaviour by managing drinking context	Long-term aim to change drinking cultures, promoting the benefits of responsible drinking and discouraging harmful drinking
Brief interventions	
Health education on controlled drinking in educational institutions	
Providing shelters for homeless drinkers and intoxicated individuals	

and clubs). These approaches have broadened the sphere of interest in alcohol-related harms to include social nuisance and public order problems (IHRA 2003). Examples and benefits of the alcohol harm reduction approach are presented in Table 16.6.

Examples of alcohol harm reduction in practice include (IHRA 2003):

■ 'Designated driver' schemes to reduce drinking and driving.
■ Improving public transport in the evenings to reduce drinking and driving.
■ Serving alcohol in shatterproof glass or plastic cups in order to prevent injuries.
■ Training bar staff to serve alcohol responsibly.
■ Promoting the safer design of drinking environments (such as bars).
■ Brief interventions advising people on moderate or controlled drinking.
■ Providing shelters for homeless drinkers (known as 'wet centres').
■ Providing shelters for heavily intoxicated individuals (known as 'sobering-up centres').

Harm reduction in drugs

In the drug field, harm reduction programmes include information about safer drug use and safer sex, needle exchanges schemes (pharmacy-based needle exchange or other forms of needle exchange), programmes to reduce the risk associated with HIV and hepatitis, and the supervision of the consumption of methadone or other opiate substitutes. Harm reduction advice about safer drug use is presented in Table 16.7.

Table 16.7 Harm reduction advice for safer drug use.

Safer places to use drugs	▪ Taking drugs with friends is safer than doing it alone ▪ Avoid using drugs in isolated places (e.g. toilets, derelict buildings, canal banks, railway lines)
Safer methods of taking drugs	▪ Swallowing, smoking or inhaling drugs is safer than injecting
Risks of injecting drugs	▪ Overdose ▪ Infection ▪ Abscesses ▪ Blood clots (thromboses) ▪ Blood poisoning (septicaemia) ▪ Gangrene ▪ Death
If you intend to inject drugs	▪ Help and advice is available from your local needle and syringe exchange ▪ It is safer *not* to inject ▪ It is more dangerous to inject in big veins like the groin or neck
Sharing needles, syringes, filters, spoons and water should always be avoided to reduce the risk of HIV, hepatitis B and C transmission	▪ Ask your GP about hepatitis B vaccination ▪ Do not use other people's 'wash outs' ▪ It is not just the needle that is dangerous, everything that is used for injecting could pass on the virus
Hygiene	▪ It is very important when injecting drugs to always remember to use clean, preferably new, equipment and make sure your hands and the injection site are clean
Mixing drugs	▪ Avoid cocktails of drugs — mixing drugs makes it more difficult to predict what will happen and for how long
Combining alcohol and drugs	▪ Can lead to respiratory depression ▪ May choke on your vomit ▪ Accidental overdoses and deaths

Source: adapted from Nottingham Alcohol and Drug Team. *Problem Drug Use: a guide to management in general practice.* Nottingham Alcohol and Drug Team, Wells Road Centre, Nottingham.

The first principle of reducing harm involves drawing attention to technique-specific hazards (related to the technology of injecting and sharing of equipment) (Rassool 2009). For example, one important initiative in the harm reduction approach has been the implementation of needle syringe schemes that provide sterile equipment, information on safer injecting and other services to people who are usually using illegal drugs. The procedure of safer injecting and methods of cleaning injecting equipment are presented in Table 16.8.

Table 16.8 Harm reduction advice for injecting drug users.

Safer injecting use	Method for cleaning injecting equipment
■ Always inject with the blood flow ■ Rotate injection sites ■ Use sterile, new injecting equipment, with the smallest bore needle possible ■ Avoid the neck, groin, breast, feet and hand veins ■ Mix powders with sterile water and filter the solution before injecting ■ Always dispose of equipment safely (either in a bin provided or by placing the needle inside the syringe and placing both inside a drinks can) ■ Avoid injecting into infected areas ■ Do not inject into swollen limbs, even if the veins appear to be distended ■ Poor veins indicate a poor technique. Try to see what is going wrong ■ Do not inject on your own ■ Learn basic principles of first aid and cardiopulmonary resuscitation in order that you may help friends at times of crisis	1 Pour bleach into one cup (or bottle) and water into another 2 Draw bleach up with the dirty needle and syringe 3 Expel bleach into a sink 4 Repeat steps 2 and 3 5 Draw water up through the needle and syringe 6 Expel water into a sink 7 Repeat steps 5 and 6 at least two or three times

Source: Department of Health (1999) *Drug Misuse and Dependence: guidelines on clinical management*. HMSO, London.

Harm reduction in tobacco

Tobacco harm reduction is a policy or strategy for tobacco users who cannot or will not stop that explicitly includes the continued use of tobacco or nicotine and is designed to reduce the health effects of tobacco use (IHRA 2006). According to the International Harm Reduction Association (IHRA 2006), examples of harm reduction interventions could include using potentially reduced-exposure products (PREPs), reduced consumption, switching to long-term nicotine replacement therapy (NRT), switching to smokeless tobacco products, and using replacement products for temporary abstinence. Currently, the tobacco harm reduction strategy is based on supply and demand reduction strategies (Esson & Leeder 2005). Advising cigarette smokers who cannot give up smoking to use oral tobacco could be an efficient way to reduce harm related to nicotine addiction (Fagerström & Schildt 2003).

Table 16.9 Prevention of HIV among injecting drug users: core package of interventions.

■ Availability of and referral to a variety of drug treatment options
■ Substitution therapy such as methadone maintenance therapy
■ Sterile needle and syringe access and disposal programmes
■ Outreach programmes and community-based interventions
■ Primary health care, such as hepatitis B vaccination and abscess and vein care
■ Prevention of sexual transmission among drug users and their partners, including access to condoms
■ Prevention and treatment of other sexually transmitted infections (STIs)
■ Voluntary confidential counselling and HIV testing (VCT)
■ Access to AIDS (acquired immune deficiency syndrome) treatment for injecting drug users
■ Provision of information, advice and education about HIV, other diseases and sexual and reproductive health
■ Access to affordable clinical and home-based care, essential legal and social services, psychosocial support and counselling services

Source: adapted from Cabinet Office (2005) *Harm Reduction: tackling drug use and HIV in the developing world.* Department for International Development, London.

Harm reduction in HIV and blood-borne infections

The aims of harm reduction strategies are to reduce the health and social harms of drug injecting and to prevent HIV transmission among injecting drug users. A core package of interventions includes exchange syringe schemes, methadone maintenance, hepatitis vaccination, safer sexual practice, improved sexual health, access to drug and HIV treatment, and clinical and home-based care (Cabinet Office 2005). A comprehensive list is provided in Table 16.9.

Needle exchange schemes

The World Health Organization (WHO 2004) report stated that there is evidence to suggest that providing access to and encouraging utilisation of sterile needles and syringes for people who inject drugs is now generally considered to be a fundamental component of any comprehensive and effective HIV-prevention programme. Syringe exchange schemes provide paraphernalia (e.g. syringe, citric and vitamin C sachets, water ampoules, stericups, sterifilts), educational resources (e.g. safer drug use, safer sexual practice, avoiding overdose, first aid) and health interventions to enable injecting drug users to protect themselves and their communities through safer injection practices and harm reduction methods. Strategies should be developed to focus on young people who are occasional or recreational users as they are often missed. In some countries, there is provision of syringe dispensing machines and mobile vans as part of the needle exchange schemes. A more recent technological innovation is the 'nevershare syringe' designed for injecting drug users with plungers in a range of colours to reduce accidental sharing.

Summary of key points

- Every encounter with a patient affords an opportunity to transmit knowledge about health care and harm reduction in relation to tobacco smoking, alcohol, psychoactive drugs and sexual health.
- Prevention activities have been viewed as existing on three levels: primary, secondary and tertiary.
- Alcohol and drug policies are now part of hospital policies.
- The importance of promoting the rational use of psychoactive drugs has been recognised.
- Harm reduction means trying to reduce the harm that people do to themselves, or other people, from their substance use.
- Harm reduction can work alongside approaches that aim for reductions in drug, alcohol and tobacco consumption.
- Harm reduction focuses on safer drug use and safer sexual practice.
- Harm reduction provides better outcomes for substance misusers as a small reduction in alcohol or drug misuse is better than zero reduction.
- Harm reduction programmes include supervised consumption of methadone or other opiate substitutes and needle exchanges schemes (pharmacy-based needle exchanges or other forms of needle exchange).
- A comprehensive alcohol policy needs population-level interventions, which focus on the availability and accessibility of alcohol and alcohol harm reduction interventions.
- The harm reduction approach to tobacco smoking has remained controversial despite the universal use of tobacco.
- In the context of HIV and other blood-borne diseases, harm reduction strategies aim to reduce the health and social harms of drug injecting.
- Needle exchange programmes need to target occasional or recreational drug users, especially among young people.

References

ACMD (Advisory Council on the Misuse of Drugs) (1984) *Prevention*. HMSO. London.

Australian Commonwealth Government (2008) *National Amphetamine-type Stimulant Strategy. Background paper*. Monograph Series No. 69. Australian Commonwealth Government: http://www.health.gov.au/internet/drugstrategy/publishing.nsf/Content/mono69-l.

Cabinet Office (2005) *Harm Reduction: tackling drug use and HIV in the developing world*. Department for International Development, London.

Department of Health (1999) *Drug Misuse and Dependence: guidelines on clinical management*. HMSO, London.

Department of Health (2007) *Safe. Sensible. Social. The next steps in the National Alcohol Strategy*. Department of Health, London.

Department of Health & National Treatment Agency for Substance Misuse (2007) *Reducing Drug-related Harm: an action plan*. Department of Health, London.

Edmonds K., Sumnall H., McVeigh J. & Bellis M.A. (2005) *Drug Prevention among Vulnerable Young People*. National Collaborating Centre for Drug Prevention, Liverpool: www.cph.org.uk/cph_pubs/reports/SM/Q3factsheets.pdf.

Esson K.M. & Leeder S. (2005) *The Millennium Development Goals and Tobacco Control: an opportunity for global partnership*. World Health Organization, Geneva.

Fagerström K.O. & Schildt E.B. (2003) Should the European Union lift the ban on snus? Evidence from the Swedish experience. *Addiction*, 98(9), 1191–1195.

Hando J., Hall W., Rutter S. & Dolan K. (1999) *Current State of Research on Illicit Drugs in Australia*. NH&MRC, Canberra.

Harm Reduction Works (2003) *Harm reduction*. www.harmreduction.co.uk/index3.html (accessed 25 November 2008).

IHRA (International Harm Reduction Association) (2003) *What is alcohol harm reduction*. www.ihra.net/alcohol (accessed 26 November 2008).

IHRA (International Harm Reduction Association) (2006) *Tobacco harm reduction*. http://www.ihra.net/TobaccoHarmReduction.

IHRA (International Harm Reduction Association) (2009) *Definition of harm reduction. A position statement from the International Harm Reduction Association*. www.ihra.net/Whatisharmreduction.

INCB (International Narcotic Control Board) (2003) *Annual Report 2003*. INCB, Vienna: www.incb.org.

Loxley W., Toumbourou J.W., Stockwell T. *et al.* (2004) *The Prevention of Substance Use, Risk and Harm in Australia: a review of the evidence*. Commonwealth of Australia, Canberra.

Marlatt G.A. & Witkiewitz K. (2002) Harm reduction approaches to alcohol use: health promotion, prevention, and treatment. *Addictive Behaviors*, 27(8), 867–886.

Mrazek P.J. & Haggerty R.J. (eds) (1994) *Reducing Risks for Mental Disorders: frontiers for preventive intervention research*. National Academy Press, Washington, DC.

NICE (National Institute for Health and Clinical Excellence) (2007) *Behaviour Change*. NICE, London.

Nottingham Alcohol and Drug Team. *Problem Drug Use: a guide to management in general practice*. Nottingham Alcohol and Drug Team, Wells Road Centre, Nottingham.

Rassool G.H. (2005) Nursing prescription: the rational use of psychoactive substances. *Nursing Standard*, 19(21), 45–51.

Rassool G.H. (2009) *Alcohol and Drug Misuse. A handbook for students and health professionals*. Routledge, Oxford.

Rassool G.H. & Gafoor M. (eds) (1997) *Addiction Nursing – perspectives on professional and clinical practice*. Nelson Thornes, Cheltenham, UK.

Rassool G.H. & Winnington J. (1993) Using psychoactive substances. *Nursing Times*, 89(47), 38–40.

WHO (World Health Organization) (1989) *Report of the WHO Meeting on Nursing/midwifery Education in the Rational Use of Psychoactive Drugs*. DMP/PND/89.5. WHO, Geneva.

WHO (World Health Organization) (1992) *Europe. Health promoting hospitals*. Networking Documents. WHO Regional Office for Europe, Geneva.

WHO (World Health Organization) (2003) *Measuring Hospital Performance to Improve the Quality of Care in Europe: a need for clarifying the concepts and defining the main dimensions*. WHO Europe, Copenhagen: www.euro.who.int.

WHO (World Health Organization) (2004) Effectiveness of Sterile Needle and Syringe Programming in Reducing HIV/AIDS among Injecting Drug Users. WHO, Geneva: www.who.int/hiv/pub/prev_care/en/effectivenesssterileneedle.pdf (accessed 26 March 2009).

WHO (World Health Organization) (2007) *Outcome Evaluation Summary Report: WHO/UNODC global initiative on primary prevention of substance abuse*. WHO, Geneva.

17 Complex and Special Needs in Addiction

This chapter deals with a number of issues related to addiction and focuses on physical health and dual diagnosis. Many alcohol and drug misusers have physical problems related to their consumption of psychoactive substances. This area of care needs to be accorded as much attention as their alcohol and drug misuse. In the UK, there is a broad consensus on the increase in the number of mentally ill patients who misuse alcohol and drugs. Alcohol and drug problems are associated with depression, anxiety disorders, schizophrenia and personality disorders, amongst others.

Physical health

People who misuse drugs, alcohol or other substances cause considerable harm to themselves and to society. This includes physical, social and psychological harm. One area of neglect of substance misusers is the care and management of their physical problems or needs. There are many aspects of alcohol and drug misuse that have an impact on patients' physical health. It is vital that this forms part of the assessment process or discussion. The harmful use of alcohol places a huge burden on the health and social care services and admissions to general hospitals.

In a study of physical health problems among patients ($n = 315$) with alcohol use disorders at alcohol treatment agencies in six European cities, Gossop *et al.* (2007) found that 79% of the sample had at least one problem, and 59% had two or more problems. Health problems were often serious, and 60% had at least one health problem that required treatment. Gastrointestinal and liver disorders were the most common problems, followed by cardiovascular or neurological problems. The frequency of drinking, duration of alcohol use disorder and severity of alcohol dependence were associated with increased physical morbidity. Current smoking status and age were also associated with poorer physical health. Older drinkers had more physical health problems although they were less severely alcohol dependent than their younger counterparts.

Injecting drug users are at high risk of acquiring blood-borne viruses such as HIV (human immunodeficiency virus) and hepatitis C virus. There has been a recent rise in the incidence of hepatitis C virus in England (Judd *et al.* 2005). Possible explanations for the rising incidence of hepatitis C include changes in patterns of injecting drug use, greater levels of crack injection and risk behaviour in newer injecting drug users; increases in the size of the population of injecting drug users is over and above any increase in protective interventions.

There are also physical problems associated with cannabis use. When cannabis resin is inhaled with tobacco this increases the risk of bronchitis, emphysema and other respiratory problems (Taylor *et al.* 2000). The Advisory Council on the Misuse of Drugs (ACMD 2008) has reported that one of the major short-term risks to physical health posed by cannabis consumption is the impact on blood pressure and heart rate, which is similar to that caused by exercise. This can be dangerous for people with coronary artery disease, irregular heart rhythms or high blood pressure, especially if they are not aware of it. Paradoxically, cannabis can disrupt the control of blood pressure, leading to a lower standing blood pressure and an increased risk of fainting when standing up. Smoking cannabis is associated with an increased risk of chronic bronchitis and potential long-term risk of lung cancer and it has adverse effects on the reproductive system and reproduction (ACMD 2008). The effects of cannabis on coordination and concentration can also result in accidents, particularly if people attempt to drive or operate machinery while under the influence of the drug.

Dual diagnosis: substance misuse and psychiatric disorders

In the context of this chapter, dual diagnosis refers to the coexistence of substance misuse and psychiatric disorders. Dual diagnosis has gained prominence partly due to the closures of long-stay psychiatric institutions – increasing emphasis on care and treatment in the community – an increasing prevalence of alcohol and drug misuse amongst the general population (Rassool 2006a), and improved recognition and screening. The combination of substance misuse and psychiatric disorders is associated with a host of serious social, behavioural, psychological and physical problems, resulting in increased demands on mainstream services. The *National Service Framework for Mental Health* (Department of Health 1999) clearly identifies dual diagnosis patients as a population with a greater risk of stigmatisation and exclusion from existing service provision. It is stated that with dual diagnosis patients, the psychiatric disorders and the substance misuse are separate, chronic disorders, each with an independent course, yet each able to influence the properties of each other (Carey 1989).

Concept and prevalence of dual diagnosis

There is still no consensus or common understanding of what is meant by dual diagnosis. The concept of 'dual diagnosis' or 'co-morbidity' has been applied to a number of individuals with two coexisting disorders or conditions such as a physical illness and mental health problems, schizophrenia and substance misuse, or learning disability and mental health problems. Two or more substance disorders or psychiatric conditions may be present at the same time, or may occur at different times (Crome *et al.* 2009). The concepts of dual diagnosis, co-morbidity or complex or multiple needs are now used commonly and interchangeably. The dual diagnosis individual meets the Diagnostic and Statistical Manual of Mental Disorders IV (DSM-IV) criteria for both substance abuse or dependency and a coexisting psychiatric disorder (American Psychiatric Association 1995).

The prevalence rate of substance use disorders among individuals with mental health problems range from 35% to 60% (Mueser *et al.* 1995; Menezes *et al.* 1996). The National Treatment Outcome Research Study (NTORS) (Gossop *et al.* 1998) found evidence of psychiatric disorders among individuals with primary substance use disorders. In a study of the prevalence and management of co-morbidity amongst adult substance misuse and mental health treatment populations (Weaver *et al.* 2002), the findings showed that some 74.5% of users of drug services and 85.5% of users of alcohol services experienced mental health problems. In summary, UK data from one national survey and from local studies (Department of Health 2002) generally show the following:

▓ Increased rates of substance misuse are found in individuals with mental health problems.
▓ Alcohol misuse is the most common form of substance misuse.
▓ Where drug misuse occurs it often coexists with alcohol misuse.
▓ Homelessness is frequently associated with substance misuse problems.
▓ Community Mental Health Teams typically report that 8–15% of their clients have dual diagnosis problems although higher rates may be found in inner cities.
▓ Prisons have a high prevalence of substance misuse and dual diagnosis.

Table 17.1   The relationship between alcohol and mental health problems.

- There are significant connections between reported alcohol use and depressive symptoms
- People report using alcohol to help them sleep
- People drink more when experiencing moderate to high levels of shyness or fear
- Anxious people use drinking 'to cope' and are more likely to avoid social situations where alcohol is not available
- 65% of suicides have been linked to excessive drinking
- 70% of men who kill themselves have drunk alcohol before doing so
- Almost a third of suicides amongst young people are committed while the person is intoxicated
- Anxiety and depressive symptoms are more common in heavy drinkers
- Heavy drinking is more common in those with anxiety and depression
- There is a significant relationship between job stress and alcohol consumption

Source: Mental Health Foundation (2006) *Cheers? Understanding the relationship between alcohol and mental health. Executive summary*. Mental Health Foundation, London.

Relationship of alcohol, drugs and mental health problems

There is a strong relationship between alcohol, drug misuse and mental health problems. The idea that people 'self-medicate' their psychological health problems using alcohol is also very well known. The aetiological theories about why individuals with mental health problems use psychoactive substances are documented in Rassool (2002). The relationship between alcohol and mental health is summarized in Table 17.1.

Drug misusers may show symptoms such as mania, psychosis, depression, anxiety and personality disorder symptoms. This is dependent on the type of drug used, the quantity consumed and the route of administration. Psychiatric symptoms occur more commonly in drug-related problems and it is difficult to distinguish between the psychiatric symptoms and dual diagnosis. A summary of the relationship between drugs and mental health is presented in Table 17.2.

Patients with complex needs

Individuals with substance misuse and psychiatric disorders are a vulnerable group of people with complex needs. Individuals with this combination of problems often have a lot of additional difficulties that are not purely medical, psychological or psychiatric. They are more likely to have a worse prognosis with high levels of service use including emergency clinic and in-patient admissions (McCrone *et al.* 2000). In addition, they have problems relating to social, legal, housing, welfare and 'lifestyle' matters. A summary of the major problems associated with individuals with dual diagnosis is presented in Table 17.3.

Table 17.2 The relationship between drugs and mental health problems.

Category of substance	Type of substance	Common mental health problems
	Alcohol	Alcoholic hallucinosis (persecutory auditory hallucinations) Depression and suicidal ideation Social phobia Pathological jealousy Delirium tremens Wernike's encephalopathy Korsakoff's psychosis Personality disorder
Stimulant	Amphetamine	Disordered thinking Hallucinations Paranoid ideas Production of random, pointless, repetitive behaviour (such as involuntary picking and scratching at the skin) Restlessness Sleep disturbances
Stimulant	Cocaine	Experience of hallucinations (visual, auditory, tactile) Paranoid feelings Irritability Toxic psychosis with persecutory delusions and hallucinations Loss of insight (condition which usually subsides within 24 hours) Depression Sleep disturbances
Hallucinogen	Cannabis	Anxiety and panic attacks Restlessness Depersonalisation Derealisation Paranoia Transient mood disorders Acute toxic confusional state
	LSD (lysergic acid diethylamide)	Hallucinations Panic reactions Flashback (recurrence of symptoms)
Opiate	Heroin	Anxiety Depression Suicide Overdose Personality disorder

Source: Rassool G.H. (2009) *Alcohol and Drug Misuse. A handbook for student and health professionals*, p. 218. Routledge, London. Reproduced with kind permission of Taylor & Francis.

Table 17.3 Major problems faced by patients with complex needs.

▓ Increase likelihood of self-harm
▓ Increased risk of HIV infection
▓ Increased use of institutional services
▓ Poor compliance with medication/treatment
▓ Homelessness
▓ Increased risk of violence
▓ Increased risk of victimisation/exploitation
▓ Higher recidivism
▓ Increased contact with the criminal justice system
▓ Family problems
▓ Poor social outcomes including impact on carers and family
▓ Denial of substance misuse
▓ Negative attitudes of health care professionals
▓ Social exclusion

Source: Rassool G.H. (2009) *Alcohol and Drug Misuse. A handbook for student and health professionals*, p. 214. Routledge, London. Reproduced with kind permission of Taylor & Francis.

Nursing interventions with dual diagnosis patients

An assessment of substance misuse should form an integral part of standard assessment procedures for mental health problems. For further information on screening and assessment see Rassool and Winnington (2006). A useful framework for utilising therapeutic interventions with individuals who have coexisting substance misuse and mental health problems identified four stages of intervention (Osher & Kofoed 1989):

1 Engagement.
2 Motivation for change (persuasion).
3 Active treatment.
4 Relapse prevention.

Within these stages exist various cognitive approaches to the care and treatment of individuals with dual diagnosis such as harm reduction, motivational interviewing, individual cognitive-behavioural counselling, lifestyle change, relapse planning and prevention, and family education. For a comprehensive account of the application of the four stages of interventions see Rassool (2006a).

Engagement with the patient is concerned with the development and maintenance of a therapeutic relationship and building rapport. The aim at this stage is to understand the client and their views, to respond to their behaviour and language, to recognise their often unspoken needs, and thereby to develop some trust and genuineness (Price 2002). The approach with the patient needs to be non-judgmental and empathic. In the initial phase, alcohol and drug misuse are not addressed until the end of the engagement process, when a therapeutic relation-

Table 17.4 Promotion of the engagement process.

▨ Motivate clients to see the benefits of the treatment process – this requires a clear idea of what they need and value
▨ Have a non-confrontational, empathic and committed approach
▨ Offer help with meeting initial needs such as food, shelter, housing and clothing
▨ Provide assistance with benefit entitlements
▨ Provide assistance with legal matters
▨ Involve family or carers wherever possible
▨ Meet clients in settings where they feel safe. This may be more constructive than expecting them to come to services

Source: Rethink & Turning Point (2004) *Dual Diagnosis Toolkit: mental health and substance misuse*. Rethink and Turning Point, London. Reproduced with permission.

ship has been established. A guideline that helps to promote the process of engagement is presented in Table 17.4.

The next stage is to empower the patient to gain insight into their problems and to strengthen a client's motivation and commitment to change. A variety of simple techniques (Department of Health 2002) can be used for this purpose, including:

▨ Education about substances and the problems that may be associated with misuse, including the effects on mental health.
▨ Presentation of objective assessment data (e.g. liver function tests, urinalysis).
▨ Balance sheets on which the client lists the pros and cons of continued use/abstinence.
▨ Exploration of barriers to the attainment of future goals.
▨ Reframe problems or past events emphasising the influence of substance misuse.
▨ Reviewing medication and the use of an optimal medication regime.

The active intervention stage involves the nudging of the patient through the treatment journey. The patient needs to have an active involvement in formulating goals and care plan. However, if it is unrealistic to aim for abstinence it may be more appropriate to consider intermediate goals that represent reduction in the harm incurred from drug and alcohol misuse, and not focusing prematurely on complete cessation (Department of Health 2002). Interventions may include the use of pharmacological management, cognitive-behavioural therapy, social support and building self-esteem and social skills, occupational therapy, welfare advice and employment services.

Substance misuse and mental health problems are chronic relapsing conditions, and part of the package of interventions is to build the skills of the patient in the prevention and management of relapses. A number of principles and strategies of relapse prevention for substance misuse (Manley and McGregor 2006) and the management of psychosis relapses have been recommended for this purpose. This approach aims to identify high-risk situations for substance misuse and rehearse coping strategies proactively.

Summary of key points

■ There are many aspects of alcohol and drug misuse that have an impact on a patient's physical health.

■ The harmful use of alcohol places a huge burden on the health and social care services and admissions to general hospitals.

■ Gastrointestinal and liver disorders are the most common problems followed by cardiovascular or neurological problems in drinkers.

■ Frequency of drinking, duration of alcohol use disorder, and severity of alcohol dependence are associated with increased physical morbidity.

■ The term dual diagnosis covers a broad spectrum of mental health and substance misuse problems that an individual might experience concurrently.

■ The prevalence rate of substance use disorder among individuals with mental health problems ranges from 35% to 60%.

■ Individuals with substance misuse and psychiatric disorders are a vulnerable group of people with complex needs and problems.

■ Alcohol misusers may have affective disorders (depression), anxiety disorders and psychosis.

■ Drug misusers may show symptoms such as mania, psychosis and depression.

■ A useful framework for utilising therapeutic interventions identified four stages of intervention: engagement, motivation for change (persuasion), active treatment and relapse prevention.

References

ACMD (Advisory Council for Misuse of Drugs) (2008) *Cannabis: classification and public health*. Home Office, London.

American Psychiatric Association (1995) *Diagnostic and Statistical Manual of Mental Disorders*, 4th edn. American Psychiatric Press, Washington, DC.

Carey K.B. (1989) Emerging treatment guidelines for mentally ill chemical abusers. *Hospital and Community Psychiatry*, 40(4), 341–349.

Crome I., Chambers P., Frisher M., Bloor R. & Roberts D. (2009) *The Relationship between Dual Diagnosis: substance misuse and dealing with mental health issues*. SCIE Research Briefing No. 30. Social Care Institute for Excellence, London: www.scie.org.uk/publications/briefings/briefing30/index.asp (accessed 5 October 2009).

Department of Health (1999) *National Service Framework for Mental Health*. HMSO, London.

Department of Health (2002) *Mental Health Policy Implementation Guide: dual diagnosis good practice guide*. Department of Health, London.

Gossop M., Marsden J., Stewart D., Lehmann P., Edwards C., Wilson A. & Segar G. (1998) Substance use, health and social problems of service users at 54 drug treatment agencies. Intake data from the National Treatment Outcome Research Study. *British Journal of Psychiatry* 173, 166–171.

Gossop M., Neto D., Rasovanovic M. *et al.* (2007) Physical health problems among patients seeking treatment for alcohol use disorders: a study in six European cities. *Addiction Biology*, 12(2), 190–196. doi: 10.1111/j.1369-1600.2007.00066.

Judd A., Hickman M., Jones S., McDonald T., Parry J.V., Stimson G.V. & Hall A. (2005) Incidence of hepatitis C virus and HIV among new injecting drug users in London: prospective cohort study. *British Medical Journal*, 330(7841), 24–25. doi: 10.1136/bmj.38286.841227.7C.

Manley D. & McGregor J. (2006) Relapse Prevention in Dual Diagnosis. In G.H. Rassool (ed.) *Dual Diagnosis Nursing*, pp. 261–269. Blackwell Publishing, Oxford.

McCrone P., Menezes P.R., Johnson S., Scott S., Thornicroft H. & Marshall J. (2000) Service use and costs of people with dual diagnosis in south London. *Acta Psychiatrica Scandinavia*, 101(6), 464–472.

Menezes P., Johnson S., Thornicroft, G., Marshall J., Prosser D., Bebbington P. & Kuipers E. (1996) Drug and alcohol problems among individuals with severe mental illnesses in south London. *British Journal of Psychiatry*, 168(5), 612–619.

Mental Health Foundation (2006) *Cheers? Understanding the relationship between alcohol and mental health. Executive summary*. Mental Health Foundation, London: www.mentalhealth.org.uk.

Mueser K., Bennett M. & Kushner M. (1995) Epidemiology of substance use disorders among persons with chronic mental illness. In: A. Lehman & L. Dixon (eds) *Double Jeopardy: chronic mental illness and substance use disorders*, pp. 9–25. Harwood Academic, Chur, Switzerland.

Osher F.C. & Kofoed L.L. (1989) Treatment of patients with psychiatric and psychoactive substance abuse disorders. *Hospital and Community Psychiatry*, 4(10), 1025–1030.

Price P. (2002) Nursing interventions in the care of dually diagnosed clients. In G.H. Rassool, *Dual Diagnosis: substance misuse and psychiatric disorders*, pp. 148–157. Blackwell Publishing, Oxford.

Rassool G.H. (2002) *Dual Diagnosis: substance misuse and psychiatric disorders*. Blackwell Publishing, Oxford.

Rassool G.H. (2006a) Understanding dual diagnosis: an overview. In G.H. Rassool (ed.) *Dual Diagnosis Nursing*, pp. 3–15. Blackwell Publishing, Oxford.

Rassool, G.H. (2009) *Alcohol and Drug Misuse. A handbook for student and health professionals*. Routledge, London.

Rassool G.H. & Winnington J. (2006) Framework for multidimensional assessment. In G.H. Rassool (ed.) *Dual Diagnosis Nursing*, pp. 177–185. Blackwell Publishing, Oxford.

Rethink & Turning Point (2004) *Dual Diagnosis Toolkit: mental health and substance misuse*. Rethink and Turning Point, London.

Taylor D.R., Poulton R., Moffitt T.E., Ramankutty T. & Sears M.R. (2000) The respiratory effects of cannabis dependence in young adults. *Addiction*, 95(11), 1669–1677.

Weaver T., Charles V., Madden P. & Renton A. (2002) *Co-morbidity of Substance Misuse and Mental Illness Collaborative Study (COSMIC) research summary*. http://www.nta.nhs.uk/frameset. asp?u=http://www.nta.nhs.uk/publications/cosmic.html (accessed August 2005).

18 Women, Ethnic Minorities and Vulnerable Populations

This chapter focuses on alcohol and drug misuse in women, in black and ethnic minority communities, young people, the elderly and the homelessness. These groups have special needs and problems associated with their alcohol and drug misuse.

Women and substance misuse

Women's alcohol and drug misuse needs to be viewed in the context of women's role in contemporary society. They use alcohol and other psychoactive substances for a range of reasons including relaxation and pleasure. In contrast with men, drinking behaviour or drug use in women is considered to be deviant behaviour and women are more stigmatised, marginalised and labelled (Rassool 2009).

Addiction for Nurses By G. Hussein Rassool. © 2010 G. Hussein Rassool

Research indicates that women with substance use problems are more likely than men to be younger, have fewer resources, have dependent children, live with a drug-using partner, have more severe problems at the beginning of treatment, have trauma related to physical and sexual abuse, and have concurrent psychiatric disorders (UNODC 2004).

Compared to consumption levels amongst men, the number of girls and young women who binge drink in the UK has risen dramatically in a decade. The proportion of people who exceeded the daily limits for regular drinking on at least one day during the previous week was found to be 34% for women (ONS 2009). In 2007, 20% of women smoked, although there has been a steady decline in cigarette smoking since the start of the decade. Women are most likely to have drunk at home (60%) or in someone else's home (11%), whilst only 17% of female drinkers had been in a pub or bar. In 2006/07 6.9% of women reported taking illicit drug in the last year (Information Centre 2008).

Issues of alcohol and drug use

The physical, psychological and social effects of alcohol are more severe for women than for men. Women develop alcohol-related problems faster than men and many die younger than men with similar drinking problems. Compared to men, women have an increased risk of developing alcohol hepatitis, heart disease, liver disease, ulcers, reproductive problems, osteoporosis, pancreatitis, brain damage, breast cancer, memory loss and other illnesses caused by alcohol and drug misuse.

Smoking during pregnancy not only harms a woman's health, but can lead to pregnancy complications and serious health problems in newborns. There is a high risk that women who smoke during pregnancy may pass harmful carcinogens on to their baby resulting in babies with lower birth weight (average birth weight of 2.5 kg or 5lb 8oz). Smoking has been associated with withdrawal-like symptoms (Law *et al.* 2003), and a number of pregnancy complications such as placental problems and an increase in the risk of preterm delivery. Babies of women who are regularly exposed to second-hand smoke during pregnancy may also have reduced growth and may be more likely to be born with low birth weight. Maternal alcohol use during pregnancy contributes to a wide range of disorders affecting their offspring including social, emotional and cognitive development, learning deficits, hyperactivity and attention problems. The most serious outcomes of maternal drinking during pregnancy are the fetal alcohol spectrum disorders.

Drugs can be harmful to a developing fetus throughout the pregnancy but the first 3 months are considered to be the time of highest risk. During the last 12 weeks of pregnancy, drug use poses the greatest risk for stunting fetal growth and causing preterm birth. How babies respond to the drug taking of the mother depends on the type of drug taken, how often the drug is used, how it is used and the amount taken and poly-drug use. A mother taking illegal drugs during pregnancy increases her risk for anaemia, blood and heart infections, skin infections, hepatitis and other infectious diseases. Heroin, cocaine and other psychoactive substances can cause withdrawal in the newborn as well as growth retardation in the unborn baby. The problems related to drug misuse during pregnancy are presented in Table 18.1.

Fetal alcohol spectrum disorders

Fetal alcohol spectrum disorders (FASD) is a term used to describe the full range of mental and physical features seen in some babies who were exposed to alcohol before birth. Alcohol can adversely impact on the reproductive process in a number of ways, including: infertility, higher rates of menstrual disorders, a decreased chance of becoming pregnant, miscarriage, major structural malformations of the fetus, preterm deliveries and stillbirth (British Medical Association 2007). The signs and symptoms and long-term features of FASD are presented in Table 18.2.

The prevention of FASD requires a coordinated and multifaceted approach: prevention strategies aimed at the general population (public awareness and educational campaigns), selective prevention strategies aimed at women of child-bearing age, in particular those who are considering a pregnancy (screening for maternal alcohol consumption), and specific prevention strategies aimed at women who are at high risk (referral to specialist alcohol services) (British Medical Association 2007). There is no cure for FASD and the management of FASD necessitates comprehensive, multi-model approaches based on the needs of the women. The guidelines for the routine care of healthy pregnant women (NICE 2003) include recommendations on:

- The provision of evidence-based information for pregnant women to support them in making informed decisions.
- The number of antenatal appointments and what should happen at each appointment.
- The use of ultrasound scanning.
- The provision of screening for a range of conditions, including gestational diabetes, HIV (human immunodeficiency syndrome) and Down's syndrome.

Blood-borne infections

Blood-borne viruses such as HIV and hepatitis B and C are transmitted from mother to baby. There is a high risk that an infected mother will transmit HIV on to her unborn baby either during pregnancy, birth or while breast feeding. Women who have hepatitis B should have their babies vaccinated as this greatly reduces the chance of their babies becoming infected. The risk of a mother passing the hepatitis C virus on to her unborn child during pregnancy and birth is low. The risk of passing on hepatitis B or C through breast feeding is very low as long as

Table 18.1 Problems related to drug misuse during pregnancy.

Psychoactive drug	Problems
Cannabis	Causes chromosomal or genetic damage (WHO 1997) Reduced birth weight and cognitive and memory deficits (Fergusson *et al.* 2002; Fried *et al.* 2003) Risk of ectopic pregnancies (Wang *et al.* 2004)
Heroin	Low birth weight, poor fetal growth, premature rupture of the membranes, premature delivery and stillbirth Withdrawal symptoms include fever, high-pitched crying, excessive sucking, muscle spasm, sneezing, trembling, irritability, diarrhoea, vomiting and occasionally seizures Babies are often born premature, are underdeveloped, have breathing problems, have infections in the first few weeks of life and an increased risk of sudden infant death syndrome
Cocaine	Increased risk of premature delivery of the fetus, premature detachment of the placenta, haemorrhage, high blood pressure and stillbirth Cocaine-exposed babies are more likely to have low birth weight, smaller head circumference, mental disabilities, behavioural disturbances, cerebral palsy, stroke, visual and hearing impairment, heart attack and sometimes sudden infant death syndrome Babies have feeding difficulties and sleep disturbances Babies have a 'withdrawal effect' including jittery behaviour, irritability and startle and cry response to touch and sound
PCP (phencyclidine) or ketamine	Increased risk of learning and behavioral problems Withdrawal symptoms with PCP (ACOG 2005)
Methamphetamine or ecstasy	Babies of women who used methamphetamine during pregnancy were more than three times as likely than unexposed babies to grow poorly before birth (Smith *et al.* 2006) Can cause premature delivery and placental problems and cases of birth defects (Smith *et al.* 2006)
Volatile substance	Increased miscarriage, preterm birth and birth defects and slow fetal growth (ACOG 2005)
GHB (gammahydroxybutyrate)	Similar to those of alcohol
LSD (lysergic acid diethylamide) and hallucinogens	Increased risk of miscarriage, birth complications and a higher incidence of birth defects If a mother continues to use hallucinogens while breast feeding, it is possible that the drug will be present in her milk and may have adverse effects on the baby

Table 18.2 Fetal alcohol spectrum disorders.

Signs at birth	Long-term effects
Small body size and weight	Learning difficulties
Facial abnormalities	Delays in normal development
Small eyes	Behavioural problems
Small head circumference	Memory problems
Flattened face	Attention deficit hyperactive disorder
Flattened bridge of the nose	Depression
Sunken nasal bridge	Psychosis
Small jaw	Increased risk of alcohol and drug misuse
Opening in roof of mouth	
Organ deformities	
Heart defects	
Genital malformations	
Kidney and urinary defects	
Mental retardation	
Learning disabilities	
Short attention span	
Irritability in infancy	
Hyperactivity in childhood	

the nipples are not cracked or bleeding. Early detection of blood-borne viruses through testing or vaccinations is recommended. The Department of Health in England and Wales has recommended that all pregnant women should be offered antenatal screening for blood-borne viruses and antenatal tests; see *Immunisation Against Infectious Disease 2006* (Department of Health 2008), *Screening of Pregnant Women for Hepatitis B and Immunisation of Babies at Risk* (NHS Executive 1998) and *Hepatitis B in Pregnancy* (Department of Health/Royal College of Midwives 2000).

Child care issues

Many pregnant substance misusers are reluctant to contact health and social care agencies fearing that the child or existing children may be taken into care. It is asserted that a parent who misuses psychoactive substances should be treated in the same way as other parents whose personal difficulties interfere with or lessen their ability to provide good parenting (ACPC 2006). The Standing Conference on Drug Abuse (SCODA 1989) has produced useful practical guidelines for professionals working with drug-using parents for assessing risk to children. These guidelines provide a framework for assessing the degree to which parental drug use may be adversely affecting the child, including meeting the physical and safety needs of the child. The establishment of Area Child Protection Committees (ACPC 2006) and the agreement of interagency child protection procedures play a key role in ensuring that appropriate procedures, arrangements and training are in place to ensure that children are properly assessed when substance misuse by parents is a possibility.

Services for women

Generally, the provision of alcohol and drug services is seldom based on the special physical, psychological and social needs of women. Women who misuse alcohol or drugs face a variety of problems including barriers to treatment entry, engagement in treatment and long-term rehabilitation. The complex factors related to alcohol and drug misuse give some indications as to why women have been reluctant to engage in treatment programmes.

Alcohol and drug specialist services could include a number of components of treatment that have been found to be important in attracting and retaining women in treatment. These include the availability of female-oriented services, supportive therapeutic environments and non-coercive treatment approaches. The intervention strategies should include motivational enhancement, cognitive-behavioural therapy, brief therapy and treatment for a wide range of medical problems, coexisting disorders and psychosocial problems.

Black and ethnic minority communities and substance misuse

Black and minority ethnic groups in the UK are a heterogeneous group with varying values, attitudes, religious beliefs and customs that affect patterns of mental health and substance misuse. Much of the impetus for current government policy that impacts on black and ethnic minority communities comes from the need to provide accessible substance misuse services. In the 'Models of care' framework there is a specific section on black and minority ethnic communities (NTA 2002: 130–138), focusing on service accessibility and utilisation, barriers to drug treatment services, service appropriateness, the professional guidance and legal framework, care pathways, needs assessment and treatment.

Black and ethnic minority communities in the UK, especially black Africans and Afro-Caribbeans, are disproportionately affected by HIV. The rate of new HIV diagnoses amongst the African community in the UK continues to rise, and is one of the most serious challenges posed by the HIV/AIDS (Acquired Immune Deficiency Syndrome) epidemic in Britain. The HIV/AIDS epidemic has compounded the stigmatisation, discrimination and racism faced by black and ethnic minority communities and this has a direct impact on equal access to health services.

Patterns and prevalence of alcohol and drug use

The psychoactive substances misused by black and minority ethnic groups are not clearly different from those used by the white population but there seem to be preferences for a certain class or classes of substances and mode of consumption by different ethnic groups which are linked with the historical and cultural characteristics of each ethnic group (Oyefeso *et al.* 2000).

In the UK the high levels of alcohol consumption in black and ethnic minority communities, especially Irish and Sikh groups, have resulted in higher rates of morbidity and mortality than for the general population (Douds *et al.* 2003). The *Health Survey for England 2004* (Information Centre 2004) reported that amongst black and ethnic minority communities those exceeding the alcohol daily recommended limit were Irish (56% of men, 36% of women) and Sikhs, whilst all other ethnic groups drank less than the recommended daily limit: black Caribbean (28% men, 18% women), Indian (22% men, 8% women), Chinese (19% men, 12% women), black African (17% men, 7% women) and Pakistani (4% men, <1% women), and was lowest amongst Bangladeshi participants (1% men, <1% women).

The Black and Minority Ethnic Drug Misuse Needs Assessment Project (Bashford *et al.* 2003) findings showed that cannabis is the most widely reported drug used (51%) followed by cocaine (19%) and khat (18%). Heroin use is reported by 10%. Cannabis is the most widely used illicit drug amongst the younger members of black and minority ethnic communities and presentations to drug services by black Caribbeans are more likely to focus on crack cocaine than other ethnic groups (including white groups) (Sangster *et al.* 2002). Crack cocaine has been reported to be used by young Bangladeshis and Kashmiris (Sheikh *et al.* 2001). Heroin is the drug of choice amongst Pakistani and Bangladeshi males. South Asians are reported to use ecstasy and LSD (lysergic acid diethylamide) (Bashford *et al.* 2003). However, stimulants like ecstasy, hallucinogens like LSD and ice (a smokeable form of amphetamine) have been reported to be used by Indians at Bhangra (clubbing) events (Bola & Walpole 1999). Khat was found to be used by the Somali community (Fountain *et al.* 2002), Yemeni communities (Mohammed 2000), Ethiopians (Fountain *et al.* 2002) and amongst Arabs from the Middle East (Iran, Iraq, Lebanon and Yemen) (Fountain *et al.* 2002).

Smoking patterns have been shown to vary between different black and minority ethnic groups. When compared to the national prevalence rate of 24% in men, the rates are particularly high in the Bangladeshi (40%), Irish (30%), Pakistani (29%), black Caribbean (25%), black African and Chinese (21%), and Indian (20%) populations (Information Centre 2004). Among ethnic minority groups, many types of smokeless tobacco are used, particularly among the South Asian population. Tobacco is often consumed in combination with other products. Use of paan (a leaf preparation stuffed with betel nut and/or with tobacco or other ingredients), believed to be a risk factor in oral cancer, is high among some South Asian ethnic groups.

Working with diversity

Black and minority ethnic substance misusers are underpresented in treatment services due to the failure to provide equitable and accessible services, poor responses in identifying and responding to the distinct patterns of drug and alcohol misuse, and an inability to respond to cultural and diverse needs. There needs to be more explicit and overt nursing commitment to diversity and more resources dedicated to meeting the needs of people from ethnic and culturally diverse communities. For nurses, the provision of culturally competent care is both a legal and a moral requirement for nurses in the Nursing and Midwifery Council's Code of Professional Conduct (NMC 2004). The goal of nursing interventions is the provision of culturally competent care that diminishes the barriers and improves health outcomes.

In the context of substance misuse, cultural competence is the willingness and ability of the workforce, services and system to value the importance of cultural diversity and to be responsive in the provision and delivery of quality services to black and minority ethnic groups (Rassool 2006). It is worth pointing out that it is not practical for nurses to have a knowledge of all black and minority ethnic groups but they can learn to appreciate diversity and provide culturally sensitive care to heterogeneous populations. In addition to the patient's cultural beliefs, nurses must be aware of their own beliefs, practices and perceptions as these may have an impact on the care they provide to clients from diverse cultural backgrounds. The main source of problems in caring for patients from diverse cultural backgrounds is the lack of understanding and tolerance and the inability to ask questions sensitively.

Some ethnocentric health interventions are clearly biased towards the dominant culture, and mainstream counselling may be inappropriate for some black and minority ethnic groups. Unaddressed ethnocentrism can compromise nurse–patient relationships and lead to misdiagnosis, mistreatment and insufficient treatment (Greipp 1995). Gerrish (2000) has put forward a philosophy of individualised care that incorporates notions of equity and fairness, holism, respect for individuality, establishing partnerships between patients and professionals and promoting independence. In this framework individualised care entails a holistic assessment of physical, psychological, social and spiritual needs, an assessment approach that can be used across black and minority ethnic groups.

The elderly and substance misuse

Alcohol and drug misuse in elderly people is a common but under-recognised problem with significant negative impacts on physical and psychological health and quality of life. The over-55s in Britain are more likely than their European counterparts to be regular drinkers (20%) and Britain is the only country in Europe to have a statistically significant number of over-55s drinking more than 6 units per day (1%) (Alcohol Concern 2007). Older people were more likely to drink regularly, 28% of men and 18% of women aged 45–64 drank on five or more days in the week prior to interview compared to 10% of men and 5% of women aged 16–24 years (Information Centre 2007). Recent research has also highlighted that the over-60s are drinking more alcohol (Foundation66 2009). Alcohol use disorders

Table 18.3 Risk factors, signs and symptoms of alcohol misuse in elderly people.

Psychosocial problems	Medical problems	Practical problems	Physical problems	Psychological problems
Bereavement	Physical	Impaired	Falls	Anxiety
Decreased	disabilities	self-care	Bruises	Acute
social activity	Chronic pain	Reduced coping	Incontinence	confusional
Loss of friends	Insomnia	skills	Increased	state
Loss of social	Sensory	Altered financial	tolerance to	Withdrawn
status	deficits	circumstances	alcohol	Depression
Loss of	Reduced		Poor hygiene	Black-outs
occupational	mobility		Poor nutrition	Disorientation
role	Cognitive		Seizures	Memory loss
Impaired ability	impairment		Gastrointestinal	Difficulty in
Family conflict			complaints	decision
Reduced			Hypertension	making
self-esteem			Incontinence	
Reduced				
self-efficacy				
Depression				

Source: adapted from Rassool G.H. (2009) *Alcohol and Drug Misuse. A handbook for students and health professionals*. Routledge, Oxford. Reproduced with kind permission of Taylor & Francis.

in elderly people can cause a wide range of physical and psychosocial problems. The risk factors, signs and symptoms associated with alcohol problems in the elderly are presented in Table 18.3.

There is limited research on the coexistence of alcohol misuse and psychiatric disorders in late life. Older people have been found to be more likely to have the triple diagnosis of alcoholism, depression and personality disorder (Speer & Bates 1992) and to have an increased risk of suicide (Waern 2005); schizophrenia may coexist with alcohol problems and complicate the treatment of both (Dar 2006). It has been reported that there is an increased occurrence of all types of dementia except Alzheimer's disease in elderly people with alcohol use disorders (Thomas & Rockwood 2001). Alcohol is contraindicated for use with many of the drugs taken by older people.

The prevalence of drug dependence in Great Britain was four per 1000 population for tranquillisers within the 65–69 year age group, four per 1000 population for cannabis in the 70–74 year age group, and one per 1000 for tranquillisers (McGrath *et al.* 2005). However, addiction to psychoactive substances amongst the elderly is due to 'iatrogenic dependence', that is the inappropriate prescribing of psychoactive substances by medical practitioners. Benzodiazepine dependence in general can be more problematic among elderly persons because tolerance to alcohol and benzodiazepine decreases with age (Bogunovic & Greenfield 2004). Tobacco is the most commonly used psychoactive substance amongst the elderly.

The consequences of tobacco smoking occur later in life and many elderly people have chronic disease including cardiovascular diseases, lung cancer, bladder cancer and chronic obstructive pulmonary disease.

Homelessness and substance misuse

Homelessness is an increasing problem in the UK and three-quarters of homeless people have a history of, or are to, problematic substance misuse. In some cases, this actually contributes to their homelessness and difficulties with finding accommodation. Two-thirds of homeless people cite drug or alcohol use as a reason for first becoming homeless (Fountain & Howes 2002) and those who use drugs are seven times more likely to be homeless than the general population (Kemp *et al.* 2006). In a survey of needs and provision (Homeless Link 2009), 39% of clients of homelessness services in England had issues with alcohol and 42% had issues with drugs. In a study of homeless people in Northern Ireland (Deloitte MCS Ltd 2004), the findings showed that cannabis was the most commonly used drug among all types of users, with 67% of the sample having used the substance at some stage. The three drugs most commonly used by lifetime users were cannabis, ecstasy and amphetamines. However, among recent and current users, this changed to cannabis, tranquillisers and ecstasy.

The relationship of homelessness and substance misuse is complex as trends in homelessness are clearly affected by changing social, political and economic factors (Rassool 2009). Homelessness, particularly sleeping rough, appears to have a detrimental effect on physical and psychological health. Generally these people suffer many health problems related to their substance misuse in combination with poor diet, lack of regular health care and poor living conditions. Health complications associated with alcohol misuse may consist of gastric/digestive problems, gastrointestinal bleeding, skin ulcers and sores, hypertension, cardiac problems, memory loss, accidental injury, epileptic fits linked with heavy drinking or temporary unavailability of alcohol due to shortage of money, loss of consciousness, and alcohol-related psychosis (Rassool 2009).

Serious mental illness is often accompanied by substance misuse problems; around 10–20% of the homeless population have both substance misuse and psychiatric disorders. In a Home Office study, 70% of homeless people had been diagnosed with depression or other mental health problem, or had concerns about their mental health (Wincup *et al.* 2003). Risky behaviours such as poly-drug use and unsafe injecting are common practices. The lack of secure housing can exacerbate the health problems associated with injecting drug use. The lack of hygiene, security and personal organisation that are part of a transient lifestyle increases the tendency towards, and exposure to, risky drug use behaviours with implications for both the drug user and the wider community (Rowe 2005). Recently, there has been a rise in the incidence of tuberculosis (TB), and this is magnified in the homeless due to poor living conditions and diet. The majority of homeless alcohol and substance misusers do not use traditional primary health care services, but are more likely to use accident and emergency services at times of crisis or difficulty.

Young people and substance misuse

Young people use a range of readily available and legal substances, such as tobacco, alcohol and volatile substances and illegal substances, such as ecstasy, cannabis, cocaine or heroin. Many young people will experiment with alcohol and/or illegal drugs and most will probably suffer no long-term physical, psychological or social harm. However, for a small minority of young people, the use of alcohol and/or illegal drugs will escalate into addiction. A central aim of the government's updated National Drug Strategy (DfES 2005) is to reduce drug use by young people, particularly the most vulnerable.

According to the 2008/09 British Crime Survey of 16–24 year olds (Hoare 2009), around two in five young people (42.9%) had used illicit drugs at some point, nearly one in four had used one or more illicit drugs in the last year (22.6%) and around one in eight in the last month (13.1%). Cannabis remains the drug most likely to be used by young people; 18.7% used cannabis in the last year. Recent trends in the types of drugs used show that between 2007/08 and 2008/09 there was an increase in last-year use of cocaine powder (from 5.1% to 6.6%) and ketamine (from 0.9% to 1.9%). Last-year use of methadone, and hence opiates, fell. Currently, 20 000 young people are receiving specialist substance misuse treatment. Five per cent are experiencing problems with dependence on class A drugs, and 90% are experiencing problems with cannabis and/or alcohol use (NTA 2007).

There is not one single factor that predisposes young people to substance misuse, rather there are multiple risk factors which act together on any one individual and contribute to their decision to use alcohol or drugs. There is evidence to suggest that the number of risk factors that a person is exposed to is a predictor of drug use, regardless of what those particular risk factors are; the more risk factors there are, the greater the likelihood of drug use (Home Office 2007). The reasons for using, and motivations for not using, drugs are presented in Table 18.4.

Presenting features

The presentation of features of substance misuse in young people may be divided into physical, psychological and social features but the patient will usually present with a mixture of these (Table 18.5).

This task of recognition and accurate diagnosis of alcohol and drug misuse in young people is made more difficult because of the increasing trend of poly-drug use. So far there have been no specialist substance misuse services developed specifically for young people, but instead they tend to be seen either by child psychiatry services or adult substance misuse services. Young vulnerable people who use substances, whether drugs and/or alcohol, are heterogeneous and it

Table 18.4 Reasons for using and not using drugs.

Reasons for using drugs	Motivations for not using drugs
▪ Escape from problems ▪ Alleviate boredom ▪ For the 'buzz' ▪ Feel more confident ▪ Ease physical pain ▪ Look 'hard'	*Relating to lifestyle aspirations and relationships:* ▪ Other people's disapproval ▪ Legal consequences ▪ Role as parent ▪ Career aspirations *Relating to practicalities of being a user:* ▪ Availability of time ▪ Financial cost *Relating to physical and psychological effects of drugs:* ▪ Personal experiences with drugs ▪ Current health conditions/difficulties ▪ Fear of effect on health ▪ Fear of addiction ▪ Fear of losing control *Relating to some perceived benefits of using drugs:* ▪ Sources of 'buzz' ▪ Sources of support/coping mechanisms

Source: Home Office (2007) *Identifying and Exploring Young People's Experiences of Risk, Protective Factors and Resilience to Drug Use.* Home Office Development and Practice Reports. Home Office, London.

Table 18.5 Presenting features of substance misuse in young people: physical, social and psychological features.

Physical	Social	Psychological
Respiratory symptoms caused by smoking Peri-oral and peri-nasal lesions caused by inhalation or snorting Physical injuries incurred during intoxication Agitation after poly-drug or prolonged use Needle tracks, thrombosis or abscesses owing to intravenous use Withdrawal syndromes	Deteriorating educational performance Family conflict Crime: petty associated with intoxication; theft to provide funds; 'dealing' as part of more serious association with drug culture	Mood changes Confusion Depression on withdrawal of stimulants Irritability as part of withdrawal syndrome Deliberate self-harm or suicide attempt Psychosis

Source: WHO (World Health Organization) (2003–4) *Substance Misuse in Young People.* WHO, Geneva. Reproduced with kind permission of the World Health Organization.

would be counterproductive to ignore their diversity (Epling & McGregor 2006). Preventive and educational programmes are of the utmost importance, as well as skills of identification and assessment strategies, brief intervention techniques, family work and social skills training (e.g. helping young people, through discussion and role play, to make informed choices and to be assertive when confronted with offers of drugs or peer pressure).

Summary of key points

■ Women's alcohol consumption, particularly in younger and older women, has been increasing over the last few decades.

■ The most serious outcome of maternal drinking during pregnancy is fetal alcohol spectrum disorders (FASD).

■ Smoking during pregnancy not only harms a woman's health, but can lead to pregnancy complications and serious health problems in newborns.

■ Blood-borne viruses such as HIV and hepatitis B and C can be transmitted from mother to baby.

■ Women who misuse alcohol or drugs face a variety of barriers including those to treatment entry, to engagement in treatment and to long-term rehabilitation.

■ Black and minority ethnic communities in the UK are a heterogeneous group.

■ Cannabis is the most widely used illicit drug amongst the younger members of black and minority ethnic communities.

■ Cocaine was reported as a main drug of use by black Caribbean and South Asian drug users.

■ Among ethnic minority groups, many types of smokeless tobacco are used, particularly among the South Asian population.

■ Black Africans and Afro-Caribbeans are disproportionately affected by HIV.

■ Cultural competence describes an ability to meet the needs of diverse communities.

■ Health and social care professionals must be aware of their own beliefs, practices and perceptions as these may have an impact on the care they provide to clients from diverse cultural backgrounds.

■ Alcohol and drug misuse in elderly people are common but may be largely under-diagnosed and under-treated.

■ Alcohol use disorders in elderly people can cause a wide range of physical and psychosocial problems.

■ Tobacco is the most commonly used psychoactive substance amongst the elderly.

■ The nature and pattern of alcohol and drug misuse in older people and the associated psychological and physical co-morbidities are different to those found in younger populations.

■ Drug misusers are seven times more likely to be homeless than the general population.

■ Substance misuse in young people ranges from readily available and legal substances such as tobacco, alcohol and volatile substances and illicit substances such as ecstasy, cannabis, cocaine or heroin.

■ Substance misuse in young people should be considered in the context of 'normal' adolescent risk-taking behaviour and experimentation.

■ There is not a single factor that predisposes young people to substance misuse, rather there are multiple risk factors which act together on any one individual and contribute to their decision to use alcohol or drugs.

References

ACOG (American College of Obstetricians and Gynecologists) (2005) *Your Pregnancy and Birth*, 4th edn. ACOG, Washington, DC.

ACPC (Area Child Protection Committees) (2006) *Regional Policy and Procedures*. Department of Health, Social Services and Public Safety, Northern Ireland: www.dhsspsni.gov.uk/index/hss/child_care/child_protection/child_protection_guidance.htm (accessed 10 August 2009).

Alcohol Concern (2007) *Alcohol and the Elderly*. Fact Sheet. Alcohol Concern, London.

Bashford J., Buffin J. & Patel K. (2003) *The Department of Health's Black and Minority Ethnic Drug Misuse Needs Assessment Project. Part 2. The findings*. Centre for Ethnicity and Health, Faculty of Health, University of Central Lancashire, Preston, UK: www.uclan.ac.uk/facs/health/ethnicity/reports/documents/rep2comeng2.pdf.

Bola M. & Walpole T. (1999) *Drugs Information and Communication Needs among South Asians in Crawley. Executive summary*. Youth Action Crawley, Crawley, UK.

Bogunovic O.J. & Greenfield S.F. (2004) Practical geriatrics: use of benzodiazepines among elderly patients. *Psychiatric Services*, 55(3), 233–235.

British Medical Association (2007) *Fetal Alcohol Spectrum Disorders. A guide for health professionals*. BMA Board of Science, London.

Dar K. (2006) Alcohol use disorders in elderly people: fact or fiction? *Advances in Psychiatric Treatment*, 12, 173–181.

Deloitte MCS Ltd (2004) *Research into Homelessness and Substance Misuse*. Deloitte MCS Ltd, Belfast.

Department of Health (2008) *Immunisation Against Infectious Disease 2006*. Department of Health, London.

Department of Health/Royal College of Midwives (2000) *Hepatitis B in Pregnancy. Information for midwives*. Department of Health, London.

DfES (Department of Education and Skills) (2005) *Every Child Matters: young people and drugs*. DfES Publications, Nottingham: www.everychildmatters.gov.uk.

Douds A.C., Cox M.A., Iqbal T.H. & Cooper B.T. (2003) Ethnic differences in cirrhosis of the liver in a British city: alcoholic cirrhosis in South Asian men. *Alcohol and Alcoholism*, 38(2), 148–150.

Epling M. & McGregor J. (2006) Vulnerable young people and substance misuse. In G.H. Rassool (ed.) *Dual Diagnosis Nursing*, pp. 97–106. Blackwell Publishing, Oxford.

Fergusson D.M., Horwood L.J. & Northstone K. (2002) Maternal use of cannabis and pregnancy outcome. *British Journal of Gynaecology*, 109(1), 21–27.

Foundation66 (2009) *Foundation66 highlights epidemic of late-onset drinking*. Press release 14 July 2009. http://www.foundation66.org.uk/news.php/5/press-release-foundation66-highlights-epidemic-of-late-onset-drinking.

Fountain J., Bashford J., Underwood S., Khurana J., Winters, M., Patel K. & Carpentier C. (2002) Update and complete the analysis of drug use, consequences and correlates amongst minorities. Cited in NTA (National Treatment Agency) (2003) *Black and Minority Ethnic Communities: a review of the literature on drug use and related service provision*. NTA Publications, London.

Fountain J. & Howes S. (2002) *Home and Dry. Homelessness and substance use*. National Addiction Centre, London.

Fried P.A., Watkinson B. & Gray R. (2003) Differential effects on cognitive functioning in 13- to 16-year-olds prenatally exposed to cigarettes and marihuana. *Neurotoxicology and Teratology*, 25(10), 427–436.

Gerrish K. (2000) Individualised care: its conceptualisation and practice within a multiethnic society. *Journal of Advanced Nursing*, 32(1), 91–99.

Greipp M.E. (1995) Culture and ethics: a tool for analysing the effects of biases on the nurse–patient relationship. *Nursing Ethics*, 2(3), 211–221.

Hoare J. (2009) *Drug Misuse Declared: findings from the 2008/09 British Crime Survey, England and Wales.* Home Office, London: http://www.homeoffice.gov.uk/rds/pdfs09/hosb1209.pdf

Home Office (2007) *Identifying and Exploring Young People's Experiences of Risk, Protective Factors and Resilience to Drug Use.* Home Office Development and Practice Reports. Home Office, London.

Homeless Link (2009) *Survey of Needs and Provision (SNAP).* Homeless Link, London: http://www.homeless.org.uk/policyandinfo/research/mapping/SNAP2.

Information Centre (2004) *Health Survey for England 2004. The health of minority ethnic groups.* Information Centre, Leeds.

Information Centre (2007) *Statistics on Alcohol 2007.* Information Centre, Leeds: http://www.ic.nhs.uk.

Information Centre (2008) *Statistics on Drug Misuse: England, 2008.* Information Centre, Leeds: www.ic.nhs.uk/webfiles/publications/Drugmisuse08/Statistics%20on%20Drug%20Misuse%202008%20final%20format%20v12.pdf (accessed 20 June 2009).

Kemp P., Neale J. & Robertson M. (2006) Homelessness amongst problem drug users: prevalence, risk factors and trigger events. *Health and Social Care in the Community*, 14(4), 319–328.

Law K.L., Stroud L.R. LaGasse L.L., Niaura R., Liu J. & Lester B.M. (2003) Smoking during pregnancy and newborn neurobehavior. *Pediatrics*, 111(6), 1318–1323.

McGrath A., Crome P. & Crome I.B. (2005) Substance misuse in the older population. *Postgraduate Medical Journal*, 81(954), 228–231.

Mohammed S. (2000) *A Gob Full of Khat: a study of contemporary khat use in Toxteth, Liverpool.* Avaanca Publications, London.

NHS Executive (1998) *Screening of Pregnant Women for Hepatitis B and Immunisation of Babies at Risk.* HSC 1998/127. Department of Health, London.

NICE (National Institute for Health and Clinical Excellence) (2003) *Antenatal Care: routine care for the healthy pregnant woman.* Clinical Guidelines No. CG006. London: www.nice.org.uk/CG006 (accessed 26 August 2009).

NMC (Nursing and Midwifery Council) (2004) *The NMC Code of Professional Conduct: standards for conduct, performance and ethics.* NMC, London: www.nmc-uk.org (accessed 28 September 2008).

NTA (National Treatment Agency) (2002) *Models of Care for Treatment of Adult Drug Misusers, Part 2.* NTA Publications, London: www.nta.nhs.uk.

NTA (National Treatment Agency) (2007) *New era for young people's substance misuse treatment.* Media release 31 July 2007. NTA, London.

ONS (Office of National Statistics) (2009) *Smoking and Drinking among Adults 2007/Drinking: adults' behaviour and knowledge in 2008.* ONS, London: www.statistics.gov.uk/pdfdir/ghs0109.pdf.

Oyefeso A., Ghodse H., Keating A., Annan J., Phillips T., Pollard M. & Nash P. (2000) *Drug Treatment Needs of Black and Minority Ethnic Residents of the London Borough of Merton.* ARAC Monograph Series on Ethnic Minority Issues. Addictions Resource Agency for Commissioners, London.

Rassool G.H. (2006) Black and ethnic minority communities: substance misuse and mental health: whose problems anyway. In G.H. Rassool (ed.) *Dual Diagnosis Nursing*, pp. 81–96. Blackwell Publishing, Oxford.

Rassool G.H. (2009) *Alcohol and Drug Misuse. A handbook for student and health professionals.* Routledge, Oxford.

Rowe J. (2005) Laying the foundations: addressing heroin use among the 'street homeless'. *Drugs: Education, Prevention and Policy*, 12(1), 47–59.

Sangster D., Shiner M., Sheikh N. & Patel K. (2002) *Delivering Drug Services to Black and Minority Ethnic Communities*. DPAS/P16. Home Office Drug Prevention and Advisory Service, London: www.drugs.gov.uk.

SCODA (Standing Conference on Drug Abuse) (1989) *Drug Using Parents and their Children: the second report of the National Local Authority Forum on Drug Abuse in conjunction with SCODA*. Association of Metropolitan Authorities, London.

Sheikh N., Fountain J., Bashford J. & Patel K. (2001) *A Review of Current Drug Service Provision for Black and Minority Ethnic Communities in Bedfordshire. Final report to Bedfordshire Drug Action Team, August 2001*. Centre for Ethnicity and Health, Faculty of Health, University of Central Lancashire, Preston, UK.

Smith L.M., LaGasee L.L., Derauf C. *et al.* (2006) The Infant Development, Environment, and Lifestyle Study: effects of prenatal methamphetamine exposure, polydrug exposure, and poverty on intrauterine growth. *Pediatrics*, 118(3), 1149–1156.

Speer D.C. & Bates, K. (1992) Comorbid mental and substance disorders among older psychiatric patients. *Journal of the American Geriatric Society*, 40(9), 886–890.

Thomas V.S. & Rockwood, K.J. (2001) Alcohol abuse, cognitive impairment and mortality among older people. *Journal of the American Geriatric Society*, 49(4), 415–420.

UNODC (United Nations Office of Drugs and Crime) (2004) *Substance Abuse Treatment and Care for Women*. UNODC, Vienna: www.unodc.org.

Waern M. (2005) Alcohol dependence and misuse in elderly suicides. *Postgraduate Medical Journal*, 81, 228–231.

Wang H., Gou Y., Wang D. *et al.* (2004) Aberrant cannabinoid signalling impairs oviductal transport of embryos. *Nature Medicine*, 10(10), 1074–1080.

WHO (World Health Organization) (1997) *Cannabis: a health perspective and research agenda*. WHO Division of Mental Health and Prevention of Substance Abuse, Geneva.

WHO (World Health Organization) (2003–4) *Substance Misuse in Young People*. WHO, Geneva.

Wincup E., Buckland G. & Bayliss R. (2003) *Youth Homelessness and Substance Use. Report to the Drugs and Alcohol Research Unit*. Home Office Research Study No. 258. Home Office Research, Development and Statistics Directorate, London.

Index
